Plant-Base

CW00865374

Discover a New Level of Health Few Will Ever Experience

Thomas Rohmer

Disclaimer:

This guide has been created for informational and reference purposes only. The author, publisher, and any other affiliated parties cannot be held in any way accountable for any personal injuries or damage allegedly resulting from the information contained herein, or from any misuse of such guidance. Although strict measures have been taken to provide accurate information, the parties involved with the creation and publication of this guide take no responsibility for any issues that many arise from alleged discrepancies contained herein. It is strongly recommended that you consult a physician, personal trainer, and nutritionist prior to commencing this or any other workout or diet plan. This guide is not a substitute for professional personal guidance from a qualified medical professional. If you feel pain or discomfort at any point during exercises contained herein, cease the activity immediately and seek medical guidance.

Before You Begin:

Bonus Gift: Free Hollywood Training Program

As thanks for picking up this book, I'd love to give you a free gift exclusive to my readers!

It's a workout program designed to get you a body like the Hollywood actors you see in movies.

With this book you'll have the nutrition side of things down pat, but to build your best body, you'll need to workout as well. And this workout will help get rid of all of the guesswork.

You'll also be the first to know when I publish new books, so sign up if you're interested in that as well!

Visit the link below to download your free workout and stay up-to-date with my latest books!

http://rohmerfitness.com/zacefronbaywatch

Table of Contents

Introduction:

We are living our lives today completely out of whack. Over two thirds of the American population is either overweight or obese (1). And over 600,000 Americans die each year due to cardiovascular disease (2). We've become more sedentary, and we rely on fast food restaurants and processed junk food to keep us full.

Our ancestors from the hunter and gatherer days would be ashamed. Back then, they didn't have too many options for what they could and couldn't eat so they were forced to stick to the basics such as fruits and vegetables. We need to get back to those roots of eating more natural foods that this planet has provided us for thousands of years. Sure, in modern society it won't be easy with all of the temptations that face us everywhere we go, but it'll be worth it.

Most people who go on a diet fail shortly after starting. This happens because people want a quick fix to looking and feeling better. News flash—there is no shortcut to your long-term health. The sooner you realize this the better. It will require a conscious effort to get and stay healthy day-in and day-out. It will be more difficult at certain times than others. However, going into it, **if you understand and accept the responsibility that *you* are solely responsible for your health and how you look and feel, you will set yourself up for long-term success.**

Once you've made up your mind on this, you need a roadmap. You need something that will be able to help guide you to the promised land of health and unwavering energy.

Sadly, most people are given the wrong roadmap, and they end up going to a place where they didn't want to go. I don't want to set you up to fail before you've even begun. That's why I'm going to provide you with a great map, which is the plant-based diet.

This is the perfect nutrition plan to help get you back to amazing health and feeling more vibrant than you ever have before. And in this book, you'll learn everything you need to know about the plant-based diet to get started with it as soon as you finish reading this book. In the following pages, here are a few of the things you'll discover:

- What the plant-based diet is.
- How to set-up and get started with you own plant-based diet.
- All of the amazing health benefits of the plant-based diet.
- Why you shouldn't forget about exercise with simple routines to follow.

Let's dive right in and get started!

Chapter 1: Why You Need to Take Responsibility for Your Health

Have you ever eaten a meal before that consisted mostly of sugar and junk food? How did you feel afterwards? I know for myself, whenever I eat a bunch of sugary foods at parties, I feel pretty bad afterwards! Compare that feeling to how you feel after completing a workout or eating a healthy meal. You feel energized, amped up, and ready to go at those times, right?

Imagine, though, if you lived your life in a complete fog. You had to drink coffee throughout the day in order to stay awake and function. You could barely walk up a flight of stairs without being out of breath. Sadly, this is how many Americans are living their lives today! Most people never realize that they're in a daze and that they could take actionable steps that would make them feel so much better and alive.

The first and most important step of any nutrition plan is to realize that you *can* change. Regardless of the decisions you've made in the past or how unhealthy you've been in the past, you can still change. You must take responsibly for your health and well being, starting right now. Nothing is going to fall from the sky and make you change. No one is going to force you to change. It must come from within you.

If your mental frame of yourself is that you're overweight and unhealthy then what are your chances of succeeding? Probably not that high! I remember when I was a kid I would see commercials for cologne on T.V. I was always impressed with the bodies the models had. I remember thinking to myself, "Wow, they were so lucky to have been born with a great body! Too bad I'm stuck with this normal body like everyone else has."

Of course, I later came to realize that you're in control of how your body looks and you're in control of your health as well. What if I carried around that same mentality today? "Oh he's only in great shape because of his genetics." "The only reason that person is healthy is because he can afford to eat clean foods and I can't."

You must begin to change the way you view yourself by changing your actions, and I get it; changing your habits and actions aren't easy. If it were easy, everyone would be in great shape. Instead, it's far easier to sit on the couch, binge watch T.V. and eat junk food.

Once you've made up your mind and determined that you will become healthy and fit no matter what, you must prepare yourself for other people who will unintentionally or intentionally try to sabotage your results.

Think about all of the food companies out there that produce junk food. All they care about is getting you addicted to their salty and sugary junk food so they can profit off of you for a long time to come! Do you think they care about your long-term health and longevity? Not a chance!

Your friends and family may get in your way as well. They probably won't understand your reasoning behind going on a plant-based diet and how it can help to improve your health. It can also be easy to give into social pressure and norms at parties when everyone else is eating freely as they please.

This is why it's critical to prep and plan ahead while on a plant-based diet. If you fail to prepare, you're preparing to fail. Think of how easy it would be to get tempted to eat junk food while at a friend's house or party if you didn't prepare and bring your own meal ahead of time!

You must always remember the bigger picture and why you started down this path in the first place. Ultimately, you're the one who is in control of your own health. So don't let anyone else get in the way of that. As long as you remember that, you will stay on track and achieve your health goals.

The overall point of this book isn't to simply tell you about the plant-based diet, but to make you successful with the diet. I want to help you get the lasting results you deserve instead of fizzling out with the diet after a couple of weeks like most people do.

Chapter 2: What is a Plant-Based Diet?

When I was a kid, I would regularly get in trouble for trying to talk to my mom while she was on the phone. I had no idea who she was talking to or what it was about; all I knew was that what I had to say was the number one priority. If I wanted more juice, she needed to drop everything and tend to my needs!

Being older, I now understand that whatever my mom was doing on the phone was way more important than what I needed. I also understand that it's rude to interrupt someone while they're on the phone. However, when I was a little kid, I had no idea of that concept whatsoever. I couldn't comprehend another person's perspective, only my own. Getting more juice was the only thing that mattered to me in that moment!

The same can be said for many people and their understanding of a plant-based diet. It doesn't make sense to a lot of people that someone would start such a diet. They don't understand the health benefits that it can provide. They don't think it's possible to get enough protein or certain vitamins.

Similar to when I was a kid, they simply don't comprehend the other person's perspective, and they're likely uneducated about the diet itself. Therefore, when starting a plant-based diet, it's important to know up front that other people might question why you're on this certain type of diet. Don't get frustrated by their lack of knowledge, instead use the time to educate them on the benefits that a plant-based diet can provide.

What is a Plant-Based Diet?

A plant-based diet simply means that you'll only eat whole foods made from plants. You'll mostly be consuming foods like vegetables, fruit, whole grains, and legumes. You'll also minimize or eliminate processed foods and refined sugars as well.

The main thing is that you won't consume any foods made from animals. This means that you'd be eliminating foods like beef, poultry, milk, eggs and butter among others from your diet. This differs from being a vegetarian because vegetarians only give up meat, but they can still eat other animal products like eggs and milk.

On the surface, it may appear as if a plant-based diet and veganism are the same thing, but they aren't. Veganism isn't necessarily just a diet—it's a lifestyle. Not only would you not eat any animal products, but you also wouldn't use any animal products either.

For example, you wouldn't wear or use fur, wool, leather or silk among other things. In terms of diet, being vegan isn't as strict as eating a plant-based diet because there's no restriction on eating processed foods. As long as the foods you eat don't contain any animal products, you're good to go. This means that you could eat foods like potato chips, pretzels, soda, and French fries.

Common Myths About a Plant-Based Diet

There are plenty of myths that surround a plant-based diet, but here are a few of the most common ones:

Myth #1: You can't get enough protein on a plant-based diet.

This is definitely the most common thing people who eat a diet consisting of fruits and vegetables will hear. People associate protein with meat and think that the only way someone could get enough protein in their diet is by eating meat. There are plenty of other options you have to get in enough protein with this type of diet:

- Quinoa
- Chickpeas
- Beans
- Tempeh
- Tofu
- Hemp

Myth #2: A Plant-Based Diet is Too Expensive.

Many people think that eating healthy foods such as leafy green vegetables and fruit is too expensive. Usually though, these people want to make up excuses for continuing to eat their unhealthy diet. Foods like beans, fruits, vegetables, rice and other diet staples are not as expensive as buying meat. And some of these food items like rice and beans have a much longer shelf life than meat does.

Myth #3: You Need to Eat Meat to Be Healthy.

There is research to show that eating a plant-based diet can reduce your risk for heart disease and type 2 diabetes (3). A fruit and vegetable centered diet can also lower your cholesterol and blood pressure as well (4). Case in point—you don't need meat to be healthy.

Myth #4: You Can't Get Enough Calcium on a Plant-Based Diet.

This is another argument similar to the one about not being able to get enough protein. However, milk and cheese aren't the only sources of calcium. You can get plenty of calcium from foods like kale, spinach and figs among others.

Myth #5: You'll Be Hungry a Lot

This idea comes from people who eat meat and think that's the only way you can have a filling and satisfying meal. How could you possibly get full eating vegetables? Well quite easily, as it turns out! Many foods you'll be eating on a plant-based diet are rich in fiber, which will help to keep you fuller longer. Beans and leafy green vegetables among other foods are rich in fiber making it hard not to get and stay full!

Chapter 3: Why Start a Plant-Based Diet Instead of Something Else?

I first wanted to get in better shape when I was 16 years old. I wanted to lean down and have amazing six-pack abs. I went all in and started a ridiculous diet:

- I ate six small meals a day.
- Each meal I ate had to contain less than 250 total calories.
- Each meal had to contain less than 10% of the total calories from fat.

As you can tell, this diet was very strict; I followed it diligently for a few months. Then one day I was working out in my parent's garage in the hot Texas summer heat, and I nearly blacked out. That's when I realized that my approach to health and fitness had to change.

I needed to follow nutritional and fitness advice that would actually leave me feeling good and energized instead of worn out. The diet I was following had a few major problems:

1. It didn't provide long-term health benefits that I needed to help me feel better and energized.
2. It wasn't sustainable for a long period of time. (I crashed after only a few months).
3. And it didn't even require me to eat healthy, wholesome foods! As long as what I ate met the above criteria, I was good to go.

Most of my whole life, up to that point, revolved around eating what I wanted, when I wanted. It didn't matter how healthy the food was, if I was craving it, I would eat it! Of course after this experience, I started to realize the importance of eating natural foods.

Eating clean helps to keep your body running smoothly, instead of accumulating waste like a toxic dump! It also revitalizes you and gives you energy to take on your day like nothing else can. And these amazing healthy foods aren't hidden underneath a rock where nobody can find them; they're all around us. These fruits and vegetables have been here longer than we have.

We can easily get them at any grocery store; we don't even have to grow them ourselves. Yet most people buy junk food at the grocery store. They'll buy all the cookies, pastries, potato chips and other processed food items they can stuff their cart with! They'll drink coffee at 2:00 in the afternoon when they're feeling tired.

And sadly, if people have a breakthrough moment like I did, it still might not be enough for them to change. Of course, breaking an addiction to sugary junk isn't easy—studies are showing that sugar is just as addicting as cocaine (5)! Even with that being said, there's something deep inside all of us that wants us to be better.

Deep down, we genuinely want to improve our health and well-being. This is when we start to look for a new diet that can help us improve our overall health and fitness. And this is when things usually don't go as planned...

Why Not Start a Different Diet?

With all of the diets in existence today, why should you start a plant-based diet? The answer to that is simple—the plant-based diet will provide you with long-term health and weight loss benefits that other diets won't. Sadly, most of the diets in existence today set people up to fail right from the start!

For example, let's say you start a liquid diet where you consume no whole foods. At first, you'll probably lose some weight and feel motivated to keep on going. After a while, however, you'll start to feel groggy and irritable from not having eaten any whole foods. Soon enough, you'll crash and binge eat everything in sight, completely ruining your diet.

It's not that you weren't dedicated or didn't try hard enough—you failed because the nutritional plan you were on wasn't set up to last you forever. Seriously who could go the rest of their lives without eating any whole foods? Another popular diet right now is the low-carb diet.

Everyone is obsessing over their carb intake so much that they seem to forget that not all carbs are bad. You wouldn't consider quinoa or kidney beans to be a bad carb, but candy certainly would be. You must take the quality of the carb into consideration, instead of labeling all carbs as bad for you.

And since a good majority of the foods you'll eat on a plant-based diet will contain carbs, it's important to understand why they're good and not evil. Here are some common misconceptions about carbs:

Misconception #1: If You Eat Carbs After 7:00 p.m., They'll Get Stored as Fat

The main premise behind this myth is that your metabolism begins to slow down later in the day when you're getting ready for bed. If you eat carbs late at night, your metabolism won't have the chance to burn them off like it normally would if you ate that meal earlier in the day. In theory, this makes sense, but it isn't true.

If you're burning off more calories than you consume (i.e. caloric deficit), it doesn't matter if you eat carbs before going to bed. Those late night carbs won't get stored as fat. In fact, it's possible to store carbs as fat even if you ate them during the daytime.

This can happen when you're consuming more calories than you're burning off (i.e. caloric surplus). The caloric deficit and surplus are critical concepts you must understand to be successful with fitness. I briefly mentioned them here to illustrate a point, but a much more through explanation will be provided in a later chapter.

Myth #2: Carbs that Rank High on the Glycemic Index Scale Will Cause You to Gain Fat

If you don't know what the glycemic index scale is, it basically measures a food's effect on blood-sugar levels. The higher a food item is on the scale, the faster it will cause a rise in your blood-sugar levels. When your blood sugar levels are high, your body must release a lot of insulin to help shuttle the glucose eaten in the meal to your cells. When your insulin levels are high, your body will be burning off sugar for fuel instead of fat.

Once again, if you're in a caloric deficit, it doesn't matter if you eat foods that are high on the glycemic index. This is because you're burning off more calories than you're consuming, which means that your body is going to have to use fat (i.e. stored energy) for fuel.

Myth #3: Fruit is Bad for You

This one seems really absurd to me. You hear all of the time about how you should eat more fruits and vegetables, but some people still believe that fruit can be bad for you. This is because fruit contains the simple sugar fructose, and this sugar can be harmful to you when consumed in large quantities. However, most people are never going to consume enough fruit to make that an issue. Also, if you're in a caloric deficit, it doesn't really matter how much fruit you consume. Are you starting to notice a pattern here?

Benefits and Functions of Carbs

Now that I have dispelled some of the common myths about carbohydrates, I'm going to discuss some of the essential benefits that carbs can provide for you. Of the three macronutrients, carbs are your body's first source of energy. When you exercise, your body will burn off carbs and use them to help give your body the necessary energy it needs to complete your workout. Without carbohydrates, your body will start to run low on energy and you'll become more irritable.

If you've ever tried a low carb diet for any significant period of time, you've probably started to notice both of these things occurring. That's the main reason why I don't feel that the low carb diet is a very good long-term weight loss solution. Not to mention, it's going to be hard to go the rest of your life without eating any carbohydrate rich foods while on a plant-based diet! Another huge benefit of eating plenty of complex carbohydrates is that they are generally high in fiber.

Fiber is important for your digestive health, and it can prevent or relieve you from constipation. Fiber can also lower the risk for developing diabetes and heart disease. So if you need more fiber in your diet, look no further than carbohydrates!

Are Carbs the Real Evil at Hand?

The answer to the above question is- no. What is at fault for weight gain is the overeating of food in general because it's so convenient and easy to do. Since you're reading this, you probably don't think much about how you're going to get your next meal. If you get hungry, you simply prepare your meal or maybe even drive somewhere to buy it. With food at your fingertips 24/7, it becomes super easy to eat more than is necessary.

In the hunter and gatherer days, you had to earn your meal by killing something or at the very least walking somewhere. That's definitely not the case in today's world. If you get hungry, the nearest fast food restaurant is more than likely less than 10 minutes away. Not only that, but the food that you'll be eating at this fast food restaurant will be fairly high in calories. This overabundance and overconsumption of food is the real problem for people gaining weight, not carbs.

Why Would You Start a Plant-Based Diet?

There are many reasons why someone would start a plant-based diet. Here are a few of the motivations people find for starting their own plant-based diet:

Helps with the Environment

When many people think about going green or saving the planet, they typically think about recycling more or reducing the use of plastic. That's a great start, but what you eat can help out more than you might guess. One of the main reasons for this is because the livestock segment is the biggest producer of nitrous oxide and methane gases. Many people think that carbon dioxide is the worst gas that contributes the most to climate change, but it's actually methane and nitrous oxide.

While carbon dioxide may not be the most damaging gas for climate change, it still has an impact of course, and approximately 9% of carbon dioxide emission in the United States comes from the livestock segment (6).

Another factor that many people don't take into consideration when it comes to livestock and the environment is deforestation. Think about it—if you're going to herd all of the animals together and keep them in one

19

place, you need large areas of land for them to live on. This can make a lot of forests disappear, which can trigger climate change and destroy a lot of natural habitats for animals living in the forests.

Kind Regards for Animals

When I was in high school, one of my friends was in a youth organization that raised animals and then showed them off in competition. Depending on how well your animal would place, you would get to sell it for a certain amount of money. He raised a young pig in preparation for the competition.

After a while of feeding and playing with the pig everyday, he eventually became emotionally attached to the animal. It was very difficult for him to let go of the pig after the competition, but that's what he had to do. The pig of course was sent off, slaughtered and later eaten. He didn't eat any meat products made from pigs for a year after that happened just to ensure he wouldn't eat his own pig.

And you don't have to raise your own pig to feel sympathy for these animals. There are many meat-eaters out there who would still feel bad or sick if they watched the slaughtering of an animal. By going on a diet based off of plants, you can help save animals everywhere. To put things into perspective, this is the amount of pounds of meat produced for the month of August in 2017 (7):

- Commercial Red Meat Production: 4.63 billion pounds
- Beef Production: 2.4 billion pounds
- Veal Production: 6.4 million pounds
- Pork Production: 2.21 billion pounds
- Lamb and Mutton Production: 12.8 million pounds

As you can see, these numbers are quite high, and you might be thinking to yourself, "How can one person's diet make a

20

difference?" Well that's similar to the attitude of, "Why should I vote? My one vote won't change the outcome of the election?" Imagine if everyone thought like that. What if no one voted because they believed that their single vote didn't matter? Then all of the sudden any single person's vote would matter greatly!

Ultimately, it's not about the single vote or a single person starting a plant-based diet. It's about the principle behind it. It's about standing up for what you believe in and focusing on what you're in control of. Sure, you can't make everyone eat a diet based off of fruits and vegetables, but you can be a good living example of someone who eats a healthy, wholesome diet for the people that are around you.

They'll see how much you care, and they'll be able to tell how passionate you are about animals. They might get curious and ask questions or possibly even try the diet themselves one day. You'll never know unless you try!

To Help Improve Your Health
And finally one of the main (and most popular) reasons why you should start a plant-based diet is for the amazing health benefits that it can provide to you...

Chapter 4: Amazing Health Benefits of a Plant-Based Diet

Here are some of the awesome health benefits you'll experience by starting a plant-based diet:

1. Improve Digestive Health

There are quite a few fruits and vegetables that contain a good amount of prebiotics and probiotics. Prebiotics are non-digestible carbs that perform as fuel for probiotics. Prebiotics act in a symbiotic relationship when combined with probiotics.

Think of prebiotics as the sidekick to any superhero. Sure the superhero is powerful on his own, but the sidekick comes in handy and is even necessary to stop evil at times. Probiotics, on the other hand, are a type of beneficial bacteria that live in different organs, and their main function is to help aid in digestion.

Of course, it's great to consume more of the healthy nutrients that our bodies need. However, it's not how many nutrients you eat that matters—it's how many nutrients your body digests and absorbs that ultimately makes the difference.

Therefore, you can consume all of the healthy foods you want, but your body must be able to properly digest, absorb and use the vitamins and minerals from that food. If it can't, then the food you ate might not be as healthy as it appeared.

This is why it's critical to consume more foods that contain large amounts of prebiotics and probiotics. Here's a list of a few things you can eat on a plant-based diet that contain a healthy amount of either prebiotics or probiotics:

- Cultured vegetables (such as one of my personal favorites, sauerkraut, can you blame me? I have German heritage. And kimchi as well.)
- Kombucha
- Apple cider vinegar
- Coconut kefir
- Olives
- Miso
- Tempeh
- Kombucha

Consuming more of these types of foods will help to line your digestive track with more healthy bacteria that'll aid in absorption of key nutrients from the other foods you consume.

2. Better for Weight Loss

Studies have shown that going on a plant-based type of diet can help you lose more weight than individuals not on a plant-based diet (8). This is because by going on a plant-based diet, you'll be consuming more natural unprocessed foods. These foods are not only healthier for you, but they also typically contain fewer calories than the processed junk food that many people are eating today.

The reason for this is that wholesome foods like fruits and vegetables are nutrient dense and they have a low caloric density. Nutrient density refers to the amount of vitamins and minerals that are in a food relative to its weight. Caloric density refers to the amount of calories that are in a food based on its weight. Processed foods, for example, have a low nutrient density and a high caloric density. So not only do they have a high amount of calories, they also won't do a very good job of filling you up because of their low nutrient profile.

Imagine eating 100 calories worth of vegetables versus eating 100 calories worth of candy. You would have to eat way more of the vegetables to reach that 100-calorie mark than you would the candy. Not only that, but the vegetables will provide your body with so many healthy vitamins and minerals, while the candy will only give you a sugar rush. Finally, you won't be hungry soon after eating the vegetables, but the candy will do little to fill you up.

This is something very important to think about because it's not solely the excess calories in junk food that kills you—it's also the lack of fiber and nutrients among other things. This'll cause you to go back and eat more soon after your meal, simply because it didn't meet your body's nutritional demands.

3. Helps with Osteoporosis and Arthritis

Osteoporosis is a disease in which the density and quality of the bones in the body is reduced. Anyone can develop osteoporosis, however women are more than 4 times as likely to develop osteoporosis than men (9). This is because the ovaries stop producing a key hormone called oestrogen once a woman goes through menopause.

At first glance though, it wouldn't appear that a diet centered around eating more fruits and vegetables would be good for osteoporosis. When you think of strong bones, you usually think about calcium. In a typical American diet, people get most of their calcium from sources like cheese and milk. You can't eat those foods on a plant-based diet, which is why most people would think that this diet is bad for osteoporosis.

Upon further inspection however, there are plenty of plant-friendly foods that are high in calcium:

- Kale
- Spinach
- Figs
- Turnip Greens
- Black-Eyed Peas
- Almond Milk

Another misconception about bone health is that only calcium matters. There are plenty of other vitamins that help make bones strong such as vitamins D and K, magnesium and potassium. Eating various types of beans, leafy greens and even getting some exposure to the sun will help you get plenty of these key vitamins.

Arthritis is another common disease that a plant-based diet can help with. It's an inflammation that occurs within one or more joints and causes pain and stiffness that can worsen with age. And research is being done showing how a probiotic-rich diet based around fruits and vegetables can help with the symptoms of arthritis such as pain, morning stiffness and joint swelling when compared to people eating an omnivorous diet (10).

4. Prevention of Syndrome X

Syndrome X is commonly referred to as metabolic syndrome and approximately 47 million Americans have it (11). That's a staggering 1 out of every 6 Americans! Syndrome X itself isn't a disease; it's a collection of risk factors that increase the likelihood for heart disease, stroke, and diabetes.

Here are the factors:

- Blood sugar: 100 mg/dL or higher
- Blood pressure: 135/85 mm Hg or higher

- Large Waist: Over 40 inches for men and 35 inches for women
- High Amounts of Bad Cholesterol: 150 mg/dL or higher
- Low Amounts of Good Cholesterol: Less than 40 mg/dL for men and less than 50 mg/dL for women

You have to have at least 3 of these risk factors to be diagnosed with syndrome X. And by consuming more wholesome foods with a plant-based diet, you can help to greatly reduce your risk for developing any of these harmful diseases associated with metabolic syndrome.

5. Increase in Other Helpful Substances Such As Enzymes and Antioxidants

When you want to get and stay healthy, eating clean and natural foods is a great start, but it's not everything. You need a complete defense to help protect you from disease as much as possible.

This is where enzymes and antioxidants can come into play. Being on a plant-based diet will allow you to consume more fresh fruits and vegetables, and if you're consuming a lot of this produce raw, you can consume even more antioxidants and enzymes.

Enzymes are a substance that acts as a catalyst to bring about a certain biochemical reaction. That science-y definition probably sounds like a mouthful so let me break it down for you; enzymes enable your body to break down food particles into usable nutrients. Therefore, the more usable enzymes a food contains, the easier it'll be to digest and process. And this is why it's important to eat your produce raw when appropriate because the cooking process destroys many of the enzymes found in the food.

Antioxidants on the surface seem equally as complicated as enzymes. They remove potentially damaging oxidizing agents in a living organism. In other words—we need antioxidants to help prevent cell damage caused by oxidants. And because our bodies are made up of tons of individual cells, it's important to keep them healthy and protected.

Here's a list of some foods that contain a good amount of antioxidants:

- Kiwis
- Pumpkin
- Blueberries
- Cranberries
- Kidney beans
- Pecans
- Goji berries

Eating more foods like these will help to prevent disease and help combat against free radicals in the body like oxidants.

Find Your Why

It's critical that you find out your core reason for why you want to start a plant-based diet. It doesn't matter what the reason is; you need to have something. Think about in the past when you've had a goal and you didn't have a clear reason why you wanted to achieve that goal.

What happened? My guess is that you probably fizzled out and gave up quickly. The reason for this is because you didn't have a crystal clear reason why you wanted to achieve that goal. If you have a clear reason why, you'll persist when you face obstacles and stay laser-focused.

So make sure that you take some time to think about what that specific reason is and write it down. Having that goal in your head does you no good—when you write it on paper, it becomes real. You need to write your goal down in the present tense to make it as if you've already achieved it.

And you also need to set a date for when you'll achieve the goal by. This way you'll give yourself a deadline to work towards to help keep you dedicated. Do you want to lose weight, gain a ton of energy and be able to keep up with you kids?

If so, write it down. Look at it regularly. And if you really want to show your dedication, then rewrite your reason(s) why every night and day. Anytime you want to give into cravings or quit the diet completely, remember your reasons why and you'll be motivated to keep going forward. Here's an example of how you can write your reasons why:

Goal: I have boundless energy by March 4, 2018.

Why?

- I want to be able to keep up with my kids.
- I want to go up a flight of stairs and not get tired.
- I want to lose weight.
- I want to feel energized all day long.
- I don't want to have to drink coffee at 2:00 p.m. to stay awake.

These are a few examples, but the more reasons why that you can list, the better. And if you're struggling to come up with reasons why, simply ask yourself why to your why's. For example:

Original reason why: I want to lose weight.

Why do I want to lose weight?

Answer: I want to feel good about the way I look.

Why do I want to feel good about the way I look?

Answer: I want to be more attractive so I can go out on a date.

If you do this for each of your original reasons why, you'll easily be able to come up with 30-50+ reasons why you want to achieve your goal. The more reasons you have backing you up, and the stronger they are, the more likely you are to achieve your goal in record time. Not only that, but it'll help you get to the core of why it is that you actually want to achieve your goal.

In the example above, weight loss wasn't really a strong motivator. Feeling good about the way you look is better, but still not quite there. However, feeling more attractive so you can go out on a date hits the nail on the head! If you hone in your attention on that, you'll be much more motivated to work toward your original goal.

Chapter 5: How to Prep and Plan Ahead With Plant-Based Dieting

Being on a plant-based diet isn't the same as any regular diet that people typically do. This is because when you're on a plant-based diet, you're more limited on what you can and cannot eat. Therefore, planning ahead with this diet is critical in order for you to be successful with it in the long-term.

For example, imagine that it's your friend's birthday and he throws a party at his house. What are the chances that the food at this party is going to be acceptable for a plant-based diet? The probability isn't that high, unless of course your friend happens to be on a plant-based diet as well. Or what about when your boss at work caters food for lunch?

The point is that there are going to be too many times when you can slip up on your diet. Most people on a diet would say, "Oh it's just one meal; it won't hurt me too bad." But as soon as you start thinking like that, you're toast. Don't be like the typical dieter where everything is sunshine and rainbows for 2 weeks and then you quit when you face obstacles.

There's no way to avoid these tempting situations. You must know that these obstacles will come up, and you must be able to find a way to overcome them. Don't try to hide or runaway from them because you'll never achieve your goal if you do.

What you can do is plan ahead by meal prepping and bringing your own meal to the party that you can eat. Of course, you might be thinking, "Yeah but won't people look

30

at me funny?" or "I don't want to look like a health nut in front of all of my friends!" Trust me, I know the feeling. I remember at my 17th birthday party, I refused to eat any of my own birthday cake because it wouldn't help me achieve any of my fitness goals.

I had a laser beam focus on what it was that I was going to achieve and nothing was going to come in the way of that—not even my own birthday cake for crying out loud!

You need to be the same way in regards to your plant-based diet. If you remember your reason why from the previous chapter then you don't have time to worry about what others are thinking about you. You'll be so honed in on achieving your goal that other people's opinions won't matter.

Not only that, but you can even use social events as opportunities to educate people about the benefits of a plant-based diet. The simple fact of the matter is that most people are uneducated about the health benefits of a plant-based diet, and you can use this time to educate people who ask you about it. With that being said, here's how you can be successful with a plant-based diet by meal prepping...

How to Meal Prep with a Plant-Based Diet

Meal prepping is simply preparing some or all of your meals ahead of time. You can prep all of your meals out for the week or even a few days ahead if you like. Also, it doesn't mean that you have to fully cook and prepare all of your meals.

You could do something as simple as chopping up all of the vegetables that you'll be eating for the week and putting them in separate containers. This way when you go to divide up your vegetables for your meals, you'll already have all of your vegetables chopped up and organized.

It could also mean cooking a certain food ahead of time that you know you'll be eating throughout the week. The cool thing about meal prepping is that you can plan ahead and prepare as much or little as you're comfortable with.

Ultimately, what makes meal pepping such a time saver is the fact that you are batching. Imagine if you ate steamed broccoli 3 times a week, for example. Normally you'd have to fire up the stove, get out a saucepan, oil it, cook the broccoli, eat it and then clean your dishes—3 separate times!

With meal prepping, however, you're cooking all of the broccoli for the week at once. This way you're only dirtying up one pan and cleaning it once, not 3 separate times.

Additionally, meal prepping will also allow you to save some money! Think about it. What's cheaper at the grocery store, an item being sold in a smaller quantity or the same item in a larger quantity? The same item in the larger quantity is cheaper!

You can save money at the grocery store when you buy in bulk, and you'll be doing a lot of this when you meal prep regularly. Not only that, but because you'll be on a plant-based diet, you won't eat at restaurants as often either, which will help to save you money. Here's the exact step-by-step process you need to take to be successful with meal prepping:

Step #1: Buy Meal Prep Containers

The first thing you need to do is buy meal prep containers. You can get these online pretty cheap for around $8. The containers simply need to have compartments (for each food item), be dishwasher safe, microwave safe, freezable and stackable. That sounds like a lot of criteria, but most meal prep containers will fit the bill. Without the containers, you won't be able to properly plan and organize your food ahead of time.

Step #2: Set a Day for When You'll Prep

The next thing you'll want to do is set a day for when you'll prep your meals. For most people, Sunday works great. It's usually a chill day when you'll have time to prepare your meals, and you can even get other members of the family to help you out, if need be. If you don't want to do all of your prepping on one day, you can space it out between 2 days— typically something like Wednesday and Sunday works best. This way, you'll only be prepping meals for the next 3 days instead of 6.

The main thing is that you do whatever works best for you and your schedule. If prepping all of your meals for the week in one day sounds too intimidating, space it out. If you're usually swamped during the weekdays, do your meal prepping on the weekend and forget about it. Don't make things harder than necessary on yourself or else you'll be more likely to give up on it.

Step #3: Determine Your Meals That You'll Prep

Now it's time to figure out what meals you want to prep. Do you want to prep your breakfasts, lunches or dinners for the week? Keep things simple and easy in the beginning and don't try to do too much at once.

If you try to prepare all of your breakfasts, lunches and dinners in one day, you'll likely get burnt out quickly. Initially, pick one meal, and prep that meal for the week until you're comfortable with doing more.

Once you've determined that, the next thing you'll need to do is think about what recipes you'll want to eat for that week. You don't have to eat the exact same meal everyday of the week, but you can if you'd like. The main thing you want to think about is balance.

In one meal, you don't want to have too much protein and too little carbohydrates. I'll discuss how much of each macro (protein, carbs, and fat) you should be eating in a later chapter, but for now consider how you can make each of your meals more balanced instead of lopsided towards a particular macro.

Step #4: Execute

Once you've gotten your containers, determine what meals you want to prep and what you'll be eating for those meals, it's now time to actually prepare the meals. The best way to do this is to focus on cooking one food item at a time then if you have downtime, use it to start preparing another food item. For example, let's say you're cooking a pot of beans.

While the pot is heating up on the stove, you could start chopping up vegetables that you'll be eating for the week. Then once the pot has heated up, you can finish cooking the beans before going back and finishing the vegetables.

This cooking strategy might seem counterintuitive at first, but it works. Many people think that multitasking is the best way to get something done. People will put on their resumes as a skill that they're "excellent at multitasking", and others will think you're weak if you focus on and complete one task before moving onto the next.

However, the research shows that our brains can't multitask (12). It may appear as if we can, but in reality, all we are doing is switching back and forth between tasks quickly. This, however, comes at a cost. People who multitask lose up to 40% productivity by switching between tasks (13)!

This makes perfect sense. Imagine you're in the zone cooking a healthy meal then, all of the sudden, you get a phone call from a friend. You now move your attention to the phone conversation and then once it's over, you must remember exactly where you last left off to start again. That extra time adds up in a big way. Imagine it taking you 40% longer to finish prepping all of your meals!

Chapter 6: How to Set-Up Your Plant-Based Diet

Here's the exact step-by-step process you need to take to get started with your plant-based diet:

Step #1: Quality of Calories Matters, But So Does Quantity

When it comes to calories, many people only regard the quality of the calories as important. For example, an avocado would be considered healthier and therefore better than a candy bar. Yes, the avocado will provide your body with way more vitamins and nutrients than the candy bar ever will. However, depending on the amounts, the avocado will likely contain more calories overall than the candy bar.

This is why you must also take into consideration the quantity of the foods you're eating as well. Many people don't think that it's possible to overeat healthy foods, but it certainly is possible. For example, you could eat the following meal for breakfast:

- 1 cup of oatmeal (300 calories)
- 1 cup of almond milk (50 calories)
- Handful of blueberries (30 calories)
- 1 tbsp. of almond butter (100 calories)
- 1 slice of toast (75 calories)
- Total calories: 555

555 total calories is quite a lot. Of course, this meal would be very filling and nutritious, but it's still more than most would expect when added up. This is important to know because it's a myth that simply starting a healthy diet, such as a plant-based diet, will guarantee weight loss when, in fact, it doesn't.

You must be able to track your calories and understand how your body works in regards to weight loss and weight gain, and it all comes down to energy balance. Everyday your body needs energy to breathe, digest food, regulate body temperature, allow your organs to function, etc. We give our body the energy it needs to perform these functions through the foods that we eat also known as calories.

When we eat more calories than our bodies need (caloric surplus), we'll store some of the calories as fat so we can use them later. When we eat exactly the amount of calories our body needs (maintenance), we'll neither gain nor lose weight. And finally, when we eat fewer calories than our body needs (caloric deficit), we'll use some of our stored fat for energy. Here's an example:

Let's pretend that David's maintenance calories are 2,500 (don't worry, we'll figure this out in the next step).

- If David eats more than 2,500 calories, he'll be in a caloric surplus and will start to gain weight.
- If David eats right at 2,500 calories, he'll be eating at his maintenance levels and will neither gain nor lose weight.
- If David eats less than 2,500 calories, he'll be in a caloric deficit and will start losing weight.

So if David wants to start losing weight, he knows he must eat less than 2,500 calories per day. That's a great start that most people will never even consider. The next thing he must determine is what he eats because it does matter. The point isn't to eat whatever you want as long as you're in a deficit.

The point is to plan ahead so you know the direction you're heading and to eat high-quality foods to feel great and get healthy.

For example, let's say you eat 150 calories worth of fruit and vegetables, and I eat 150 calories from a chocolate bar. Are we equal? Well kinda. The total amount of calories we ate was the same.

There's no arguing this because a calorie is a calorie, just like a yard of wood is the same length as a yard of sheet metal. However, the quality of the calories is vastly different. The fruits and vegetables you ate will provide you with fiber, keeping you fuller for a longer period of time. The fruits and vegetables also contain way more vitamins and minerals than the chocolate bar does.

And when you're eating less calories overall to lose weight, it's important that you make those calories count. You want to be consuming high quality foods because that's how you'll stay full for long periods of time even when your calories are being restricted. Now let's move on and determine how many calories you should be eating...

Step #2: Determine Your Resting Metabolic Rate

Like I mentioned in the previous step, your body needs energy (calories) in order to continue on with all of its chemical functions like breathing, digesting food, organ function, etc. The amount of calories you burn in any given day is your resting metabolic rate (rmr). Once you figure out your body's rmr, you can then determine how many calories you need to eat to start burning fat.

Determining your rmr is simple—multiply your bodyweight in pounds by 13.
Let's use myself as an example:

Bodyweight=200 pounds
200 x 13= RMR of 2,600

This means that if I eat less than 2,600 calories, I'll be in a caloric deficit and will start to lose weight. If I eat more than 2,600 calories, I'll be in a caloric surplus and will start to gain weight. And finally, if I eat exactly 2,600 calories, I'll be at maintenance and will neither gain nor lose weight.

The question is—how big of a caloric deficit do you need to create in order for it to translate into pounds lost? There's about 3,500 calories in one pound of fat (14), meaning that you must create a cumulative caloric deficit of 3,500 calories in order to lose 1 pound. So if you divide 3,500 by 7 days in a week, you'll need to create an average daily caloric deficit of 500 calories to lose 1 pound per week.

Referring back to the example from above, here's what that would translate to:

RMR- 2,600 – 500= 2,100

This means that I need to eat 2,100 calories every day if I want to lose 1 pound per week. The more weight you have to lose, the larger the caloric deficit you can create. For example, you could eat at a caloric deficit of 750 calories and lose 1.5 pounds per week, or you could eat at a deficit of 1,000 calories to lose 2 pounds per week.

Essentially, for every 250 calories you can expect to lose an additional .5-pound. The key is to not get carried away. You might want to lose all of the weight as soon as possible and jump right into a 1,000-calorie caloric deficit.

That may not be the best idea. For most people, losing 1 pound per week by creating a 500-calorie caloric deficit is golden. Imagine yourself a year from now being 52 pounds lighter without having to put forth much effort! That's much better than spinning your wheels trying to lose 100 pounds in that same time frame.

Step #3: Macros Matter Too, Here's What to Do

In case you're unfamiliar, a macro is simply a protein, carb or fat. And now we're going to figure out exactly how many grams of carbs, protein and fat you need to be eating on a daily basis. From there, you'll simply eat that much following the guidelines of the plant-based diet and start seeing results. It really is that simple.

Before we can get into the specifics of each macro, it's critical that you know what your resting metabolic rate is by multiplying your bodyweight by 13.

Then if you want to lose weight, subtract 500 from your RMR. This is the total amount of calories you'll eat on a daily basis.

Once you know that information, you can move onto the next section.

Setting Up Your Macro Percentages

The first thing we must determine is the percentage of our diet each macronutrient (protein, carb and fat) will make up. Here are the percentages:

- Protein: 35% of total calories
- Carbs: 40% of total calories
- Fat: 25% of total calories

Now that you know the total amount of calories you need to eat, and you know the percentage for each macro, we can now determine how many calories of protein, carbs and fat you'll need to eat. Before we do though, it's important to remember the following:

Number of calories per gram of protein=4
Number of calories per gram of carb=4
Number of calories per gram of fat=9

I'll use myself as an example again:

Resting metabolic rate=2,600 calories

If I want to burn fat:

2,600-500=2,100 daily calories

2,100 x .35= 735 total daily calories from protein
2,100 x .40= 840 total daily calories from carbs
2,100 x .25= 525 total daily calories from fat

You can determine the grams equivalent of these total calorie numbers by doing the following:

735/4= 183.75 grams of protein per day
840/4= 210 grams of carbs per day
525/9= 58.3 grams of fat per day

Yes these numbers are very exact; however, don't try to be perfect. The reality is that you'll rarely eat 58.3 grams of fat spot on so don't fret over it. Instead, try to get within 5%-10% of the numbers and you'll be fine.

Step #4: Follow the Plant-Based Diet

At this point, most of the hard work is already done. You already know how many calories you need to eat and your exact macro percentages as well. From here, all you have to do is execute by avoiding any food products made from animals. The plant-based diet provides the structure for what

41

you should be eating, and the numbers you figured out earlier will tell you how much you should be eating.

Step #6: Measure and Adjust

You might be thinking, this sounds great and all, but how do I actually track and measure my calories and macro percentages? This is certainly the most tedious part of any diet, but remember what gets measured gets managed. You must track and account for the calories you're eating or else you'll have no clue what direction you're heading.

The easiest way to track your macros is to go to the app store, type in macro tracker, and download one of the many apps that will track your macros. Most of the apps cost a couple of dollars, but that's a small price to pay. You can type in the food you're eating and it'll tell you how many calories are contained in the food and how much protein, carbs and fat it has. Most of the apps even have a barcode scanner where you can take a picture of what you're eating and it'll automatically add the macros towards your daily numbers.

You'll have your phone on you wherever you go so if you eat at a restaurant that's plant-based friendly, for example, you can track the macros and calories right then and there. If you decide not to use an app, you'll have to track your macros using nutritional labels or by searching the nutritional information online. From there, you'll have to calculate the numbers yourself and record it on a note app or with pen and paper, which is certainly not ideal.

The more inconvenient something is to do, the less likely you are to stick with it. The plant-based diet is a great nutritional plan but only if you're able to keep up with it for the long haul. You want to keep things as simple and easy as possible—spend a couple of bucks and indulge in a macro tracking app to take the load off your shoulders. It'll pay for itself many times over.

The other thing you'll need to get is a food scale. You can get one of these on Amazon for around $11. This'll allow you to figure out the number of grams in the foods you're eating and calculate the macros from there.

Once you've been doing this diet for a while, you'll eventually start to get a feel for how you need to eat in order to lose weight. You'll know the general macro contents of the meals you regularly eat. You'll be able to do the eyeball test and guess roughly how many calories are in the foods you're eating.

This is a skill that'll come with time. Be patient and don't rush it because that's when you'll start overestimating your calories. Tracking everything as accurately as possible is the key to success with any nutritional approach that you do. Be diligent about your measuring, especially in the beginning, even though it's quite tedious.

It might take you a couple of weeks to get used to measuring and recording everything that you eat and drink. Be patient with yourself if it takes a few weeks for you to start seeing results. You'll get better and better with the process as time goes on. Nobody is a master at something the first time they do it.

You also might be wondering how close you have to be to hitting your exact macro percentages. The reality is that you'll never be 100% accurate with your numbers. Using the example from earlier, you'll never eat exactly 58.3 grams of fat each day and that's ok. You'll want to aim to be within 5-10% of what I recommend. For example, one day you might intake 35% of your diet from fat and only 25% from protein. It's not worth the extra stress of getting every little number exactly right—you'll drive yourself nuts. You want to generally be as consistent and accurate as you possibly can.

The other thing you'll want to do is measure your weight. One mistake a lot of people make is that they weigh themselves too often. Our bodies are constantly fluctuating in weight sometimes by as much as 5 pounds (15). So one morning you might weigh yourself and the scale says you lost weight so you're happy. Then the next day you step on the scale and now you gained half a pound.

At this point, you'd be freaking out and wondering, "What in the world is going on?" Imagine having to fight this psychological battle each and every week. Every week you have to overcome negative thoughts and worries:

- Is my diet actually working?
- Am I doing something wrong?
- Should I quit?
- Should I try a different nutritional approach?

You would have to overcome all of those doubts before you could start making any real progress. The reality is that nothing is wrong with you; the problem is that the scale is deceiving you. It's making you think that you've gained weight when in reality your bodyweight is simply fluctuating.

Therefore, it's important to weigh yourself as consistently as you possibly can. Weigh yourself first thing in the morning before you've eaten anything. In addition to that, only weigh yourself once a week. One week is long enough for you to know if the weight on the scale has gone down it's because of actual weight loss, not because of a fluctuation.

Overall, I want you to focus on the bigger picture when it comes to weight loss. Over the past 3 months, has the direction on the scale been going the way you want it to? If so, then great, you're making progress! That's what matters. Don't freak out and question everything you're doing all because you didn't lose any weight one week.

Chapter 7: Coming Diet with Exercise to Maximize Your Health

Early on when I first got interested in health and fitness, I became too focused on my training and not my diet. I wanted to improve my skills for basketball, and I thought training was the best way to achieve my goal. Sure, I'd workout hard, but my diet still consisted mostly of processed junk food!

Now I realize that nutrition is extremely important regardless of what your goal is—to become healthier, improve sports performance, build a better looking body, etc. Don't be like the opposite version of myself and only care about your diet while completely forgetting about exercise. Here's why...

It's no secret that following a plant-based diet will greatly improve your health. However, diet isn't the end all be all. You also need to be more active as well. The truth is that America is becoming more and more sedentary as a country as we've moved more towards desk jobs and other sedentary occupations, and the statistics show it:

- Over 600,000 Americans die each year due to cardiovascular disease.
- The average American watches 5 hours of T.V. a day (16).
- 80% of Americans fail to reach the recommended amount of weekly exercise (17).
- A sedentary individual averages 1,000-3,000 steps per day when the recommended amount is 10,000 (18).

Sure, diet can help to prevent a lot of diseases and keep us healthy, but we're meant to move more. We need to keep our blood flowing, our lymphatic system moving, our heart rate up, etc. Think about people who lived in the hunter and gatherer days. They couldn't wake up, walk to their fridge, take out a carton of milk and pour themselves a bowl of cereal.

They had to go out and *earn* their food. They had to hunt it down, kill it, skin it, clean it, cook it and then eat it. Every single time. Even if you were a gatherer and not a hunter, you still had to move from place-to-place collecting food.

Fast forward to the present day, and look at how most people live. Anytime you're hungry, you can get in your car and drive through a fast food restaurant to grab a bite to eat. You drive to your desk job where you'll be sitting for most of the day. Then when you come home, you sit in a comfy recliner where you can watch T.V. for the rest of the evening while you snack on potato chips.

Exercising more doesn't mean that you have to lift weights 6 days a week like a hardcore bodybuilder. It can be something as simple as going for a mile long walk, 3 days a week. Start with something simple that you enjoy doing and build on it as time goes on. The last thing you want to do is go all in and burn yourself out too quickly.

I see this happen all the time. People will want to start working out to get in better shape. So they'll immediately jump right into an intense 5-day per week workout routine. Two weeks later, they'll quit and go right back to their old habits.

If it has been years since you've exercised regularly, then take it slow and build your way up. For example, you could start with exercising 2 days per week for a month. Then once you've achieved that, you can move up to 3 days per week the following month, and 4 days the month after that.

Exercise Routines for You to Follow

Even if you favor running over weightlifting or vice versa, I recommend that you eventually do both. Weightlifting has many benefits:

- Improves bone density, which can help with the prevention of osteoporosis
- Helps with sarcopenia
- Strengthens ligaments and tendons
- Boosts your metabolism

And doing cardio also has some great benefits as well:

- Stronger heart and lungs
- Better sleep
- Helps prevent disease
- Reduces stress

Therefore, I'm going to be providing you with both a resistance-training workout you can do as well as a cardio workout you can follow. Here's the weight workout:

This resistance-training workout consists of two different workouts—A and B. You'll simply alternate between workout A and workout B every time you go to the gym. Here's an example of how to set up your gym schedule depending on how many days per week you want to workout:

If you want to workout 2 times per week:

Monday: Off
Tuesday: Workout A
Wednesday: Off
Thursday: Off

Friday: Workout B
Saturday: Off
Sunday: Off

If you want to workout 3 times per week:

Monday: Workout A
Tuesday: Off
Wednesday: Workout B
Thursday: Off
Friday: Workout A
Saturday: Off
Sunday: Off

Following Monday: Workout B

If you want to workout 4 times per week:

Monday: Workout A
Tuesday: Workout B
Wednesday: Off
Thursday: Workout A
Friday: Workout B
Saturday: Off
Sunday: Off

Here are the workouts:

Workout A: Chest, Shoulders, and Triceps

- Incline Barbell Bench Press- 3 sets of 6 reps 3 min rest btw (between) sets

- Seated DB Military Press- 3 sets of 6 reps 3 min rest btw sets

- DB Skull Crushers- 3 sets of 8 reps 90 sec rest btw sets

- Standing DB Lateral Raises- 3 sets of 10 reps 1 min rest btw sets

- Bent Lateral Raises- 3 sets of 12 reps 1 min rest btw sets

Workout B: Back, Legs, and Biceps

- Weighted Pull-Ups (replace with lat-pulldown if unable to do pull-ups)- 3 sets of 6 reps 2 min rest btw sets

- Bulgarian Split Squats- 3 sets of 8 reps (per leg) 2 min rest btw sets

- Incline DB Curls- 3 sets of 8 reps 90 sec rest btw sets

- Bent Over Rows- 3 sets of 8 reps 2 min rest btw sets

- Hammer Curls- 3 sets of 10 reps 1 min rest btw sets

This is a good workout to do regardless of whether or not you want to build muscle or burn fat. Many people try to change up their workout and do higher reps when trying to burn fat. Many people think that higher reps burn fat and lower reps build muscle, but that is a big myth. All rep ranges build muscle; they stimulate a different type of hypertrophy—sarcoplasmic vs myofibrillar.

Sure higher reps might burn a few extra calories, which might indirectly lead to fat loss, but don't rely on it. The easiest way to think about it is to use your workouts to help you build muscle, and use your diet to help you control your calories for fat loss.

What Should You Do for Cardio?

In addition to all of the health benefits cardio can provide to you, cardio is also cool for helping you burn additional calories. This means one of two things for you:

1. You'll reach any weight loss goals you have sooner.

Or:

2. You'll have more leeway in your plant-based diet plan.

Here's the best cardio workout on the planet you can do 2-3 times per week for the best results.

Part 1: High Intensity Interval Training (HIIT)

Alternate between a high intensity and a low intensity for 15-30 minutes on your choice of cardio machine. Here's an example on a treadmill:

- Run at 7.5 mph for 1 minute
- Walk at 3.5 mph for 1 minute
- Repeat for 10-15 minutes

Part 2: Steady State Cardio (Done immediately after HIIT)

Example on a treadmill: Walk at a constant pace of 3.5-4 mph for 10-15 minutes.

Note: If you need to adjust the intensity of the HIIT then do so. You can alter the run/walk ratios (i.e. run for 30 seconds and walk for 1.5 minutes), or you can decrease the intensity of each run (i.e. run at 6 mph instead of 7.5). And if what I prescribed is too easy, ramp up the intensity accordingly.

The secret to the effectiveness of this workout lies in the fact that we're combining intense cardio with slow, steady state cardio. Most people will do one or the other but not both in the same cardio session. The intense cardio will release free fatty acids into the bloodstream, and then the steady state cardio will burn them off! If you only did the HIIT, your body would reabsorb the released fatty acids. That's why you want to combine both for maximum efficiency.

Of course, if this cardio workout is too intense for you then feel free to use walking as your form of cardio. You can simply go outside and walk for 30 minutes 3 days per week. Don't worry, walking is not for the weak as some fitness enthusiasts might have you believe!

As a matter of fact, walking helps with the recovery of your lymphatic system better than intense cardio does (19). The main point is to be more active overall in addition to the healthy nutritional changes that you'll be making to your diet. Focus on the bigger picture (long-term health and longevity), and make the time to exercise more!

Chapter 8: The Secret (No One Will Tell You) to Actually Be Successful with This Diet

This book has provided you with the tools that you need to be successful with the plant-based diet. However, simply having the tools isn't always enough. Your mindset is also an essential component. Some people fail because they're using the wrong tools (i.e. following the wrong diet or insane workouts), but many others fail before the journey has even begun due to their mentality.

A common fitness goal people have is building a great-looking body. People think that once they get a killer body, their lives will magically change. Women will be all over them, their relationships will improve, they'll get a raise at work or whatever else. Few if any of those things will actually happen once you get in shape. Yes, you'll get compliments along the way from your friends and family, which will feel good, but don't expect to have your choice of super models to date.

The real prize that comes from getting into shape is the person you'll become. It takes a lot of discipline, self-motivation and persistence to get in great shape. These are the qualities you'll be developing in yourself on your journey. Once you do reach your goal, you'll not only have these characteristics deeply ingrained inside of you, but you'll also have a healthy body you can be proud of.

The self-growth and self-improvement will be the core reason why someone would become more attracted to you, or why you would get a raise at work. My senior year of high school, I scored 28 points during the opening game of the basketball season. It was an incredible feeling that I'll never forget. But what made that moment so special?

I felt ecstatic because I earned it. Nobody gave me those 28 points—I had worked hard for them by developing my skills during the offseason. I was putting in the work alone in the gym when nobody else was watching. It was never about showing off or looking cool in front of other people.

In fact, it wasn't even about trying to put up huge numbers during games. It was about doing what I loved. I loved basketball, whether I was playing in a competitive game or shooting in my backyard. I was after the process, not the prize; that's why I succeeded.

I carried this same philosophy into my fitness training and health, and it's how you'll be successful with it as well. Of course, this sounds counter-intuitive. But look around and you'll notice that most people *only* want the prize and want nothing to do with the process. That's why they fail.

Take lottery winners, for example. Wouldn't it be cool to win millions of dollars? Studies show otherwise (20). Roughly 44% of lottery winners lose all of their earnings within 5 years. They go through divorce, drug abuse, robberies, and other tragedies. Their so-called "friends" and family will start to hound them for money. The same thing would happen if there was a weight loss pill that would have you waking up with a six-pack. You wouldn't learn anything from it, and you'd quickly gain the weight back.

You must accept where you're at right now. Everyone has to start from somewhere, and it'll only get better from here. Beyond that, you must find a way to make the process enjoyable. This is the only way you'll exercise regularly and stick to a plant-based diet for a long time to come.

Finally, understand that health and fitness is a lifelong journey and not a sprint. This will take a lot of the pressure off you to feel like you have to succeed tomorrow.

Take a step back. Breathe. And *always* stay true to the process. That's how you'll flourish.

Chapter 9: 42 Plant-Based Recipes

Potato Salad

Ingredients:

- 2 cups of chopped and peeled potatoes
- 1/4 cup of low-fat (eggless) mayonnaise
- 1/2 cup of chopped celery
- 1 tbsp. of soy sauce
- 1 tbsp. of rice vinegar
- 1 large clove of minced garlic
- Dill weed to taste
- Pepper to taste
- Chili powder to taste

Directions:

1. Steam the peeled potatoes for roughly 15 minutes.
2. Let the potatoes cool slightly and chop them coarsely.
3. Put all of the other ingredients together in a bowl and mix them.
4. Add in and stir the potatoes.
5. Serve and enjoy!

Number of servings: 4

Macros (per serving):

Calories: 100.5
Protein: 1.7 g

Carbs: 15.6 g
Fat: 3.4 g

Spanish Rice

Ingredients:

- 1/2 head cauliflower, grate in a food processor
- 2 green onions, diced
- 1 tomato, diced
- 1/2 orange bell pepper, diced
- 1/2 jalapeno pepper, diced
- 1 tbsp. fresh lemon juice
- 2 tbsp. cilantro, minced
- 1/2 an avocado, mashed
- 1/2 tsp. chili powder
- 1/2 tsp. paprika
- 3/4 tsp. sea salt

Directions:

1. Grate cauliflower in a food processor.
2. Puree the remaining ingredients together in food processor until it creates a guacamole-like consistency.
3. Add in the grated cauliflower to the mixture, mix and serve!

Number of servings: 2

Macros (per serving):

Calories: 130.0
Protein: 4.7 g
Carbs: 16.1 g
Fat: 7.4 g

Energy Bars

Ingredients:

- 1/4 cup sunflower seed butter
- 1/4 cup chia seeds
- 2 tbsp. cacao powder
- 2 tbsp. PB2
- 1 tbsp. coconut butter
- 1/4 cup unsweetened reduced-fat shredded coconut
- 2 tbsp. almond flour

Directions:

1. Add all ingredients together minus the final 1/4 cup shredded coconut.
2. Press the mixture into a small container lined with waxed paper and refrigerate for 1-2 hours to make slicing easier.
3. Once sliced, coat the bars with the final 1/4 cup of shredded coconut.
4. Individually wrap each bar in waxed paper.
5. Store in refrigerator overnight, serve and enjoy!

Number of servings: 4

Macros (per serving):

Calories: 231.1
Protein: 9.6 g
Carbs: 16.0 g
Fat: 16.4 g

Waffles

Ingredients:

- 2 cups of rolled oats
- 2 tsp. of sugar
- 1 tsp. vanilla
- 1/4 cup applesauce
- 1 tbsp. of sugar
- 1 tsp. of vanilla
- 1/2 tsp. of baking soda
- 1/2 tsp. of baking powder
- 2 cups of water
- 1 tsp. cinnamon

Directions:

1. Put all of the ingredients in a blender, and blend until smooth.
2. Pour batter into waffle iron and cook.
3. Add any desired fruit, serve and enjoy!

Number of servings: 4

Macros (per serving):

Calories: 168.6
Protein: 6.4 g
Carbs: 30.3 g
Fat: 2.6 g

Protein Muffins

Ingredients:

- 30 grams (about 1/4 cup) brown rice protein powder
- 1/4 cup flax meal
- 1/2 tsp. baking powder
- 1/4 tsp. baking soda
- 1/8 tsp. salt
- 1/4 tsp. liquid stevia (more or less)
- 5 tbsp. water
- 1 tsp. rice vinegar

Directions:

1. Preheat oven to 350 degrees F.
2. Grease a round ramekin with palm shortening.
3. In a small bowl, put the protein powder, flax meal, baking powder, baking soda and salt in the bowl and mix together.
4. Add in and stir in the water, stevia and vinegar.
5. Spread into the prepared ramekin, making a thick batter.
6. Bake mixture for roughly 20 minutes.
7. Remove from ramekin and let cool briefly before serving.

Number of servings: 2

Macros (per serving):

Calories: 120.6
Protein: 15.0 g
Carbs: 6.3 g
Fat: 4.5 g

Plant-Based Taco Dinner

Ingredients:

- 2 cups textured vegetable protein
- 2 cups boiling water
- 1/4 cup olive oil
- 1 packet of Publix taco seasoning mix

Directions:

1. Put the textured vegetable protein into a bowl with the seasoning packet.
2. Add in the boiling water and olive oil and mix the ingredients together.
3. Cook over medium heat in a pan sprayed with cooking oil.
4. Cook until lightly browned, serve and enjoy!

Number of servings: 8

Macros (per serving):

Calories: 154.7
Protein: 12.0 g
Carbs: 9.2 g
Fat: 6.8 g

Peanut Butter Cups

Ingredients:

- 8 oz. (8 squares) divided Baker's unsweetened chocolate
- 1 cup chunky natural peanut butter
- 5 pitted Medjool dates
- 1/2 cup divided agave nectar
- 1/4 cup divided unrefined virgin coconut oil

Directions:

1. Line mini muffin tin with mini cupcake liners.
2. Melt 4 oz. (4 squares) of the chocolate in a double boiler over medium heat and stir frequently with a silicon spatula until melted.
3. Add 2 tbsp. of the coconut oil and 3 tbsp. of the agave nectar and mix well. Immediately remove from heat.
4. Use a spoon to spread the chocolate mixture into the bottom of the cupcake liners.
5. Place the peanut butter and dates into a food processor with 2 tbsp. of the agave nectar and blend until well combined.
6. Roll the peanut butter mixture into small, 3/4-inch balls and flatten, and press one into each cup.
7. Repeat step 2 exactly with the other half of the chocolate, oil and agave nectar.
8. Spread the chocolate mixture on top of the cups, sealing in the peanut butter mixture.
9. Place the tins in the fridge to harden for 2 hours, serve and enjoy!

Number of servings: 24

Macros (per serving):

Calories: 147.9
Protein: 4.0 g
Carbs: 9.7 g
Fat: 12.6 g

Cauliflower Macaroni and Cheese (Plant-Based)

Ingredients:

- 2, 1/2 Cups Pre-Grated Cauliflower

Cheese Sauce Ingredients:

- 3 tbsp. ground flax
- 3 tbsp. unsweetened almond milk
- 7 tbsp. nutritional yeast
- 1 tsp. melted coconut oil
- 2 tsp. stone ground mustard
- 1/4 tsp. garlic powder
- 1/4 tsp. onion powder
- 1/4 tsp. sea salt
- 1/2 tsp. Sriracha hot sauce
- Pepper to taste

Topping Ingredients:

- 1 tbsp. almond flour
- 1 tbsp. nutritional yeast

Directions:

1. Pre-heat oven to 450 degrees F.
2. In a large skillet, cook grated cauliflower until translucent, which will be roughly 7-10 minutes on medium heat.
3. In a large bowl, put all of the cheese sauce ingredients together and mix well.
4. Add in the cauliflower to the cheese sauce and stir well.
5. Scoop cauliflower into ramekins or a baking dish.
6. Top the mixture with almond flour and nutritional yeast topping.

7. Put the mixture in the oven and bake for about 25-30 minutes or until golden brown.
8. Remove from oven, let cool and enjoy!

Number of servings: 3

Macros (per serving):

Calories: 217.3
Protein: 16.3 g
Carbs: 24.2 g
Fat: 8.5 g

Asparagus Soup

Ingredients:

- One large can of drained and rinsed white beans
- 1/2 lb. of fresh asparagus
- 2 small chopped onions
- 4 cloves of chopped garlic
- 2 stalks of chopped celery
- 5 cups of vegetable broth
- 1 tbsp. of Italian seasoning
- 1 tsp. of jerk seasoning
- 2 tbsp. of olive oil
- Soy creamer to taste
- Salt to taste

Directions:

1. Chop all of ingredients and set to the side.
2. Heat the olive oil in a heavy bottomed pot then add in the garlic and onions and sauté for 6 minutes.
3. Add in the salt, jerk seasoning, herbs, celery and asparagus, and sauté for another 6 minutes.
4. Add in the vegetable broth and white beans.
5. Bring to a simmer and cook ten minutes.
6. With a hand blender, blend to a desired texture.
7. Simmer for 6 more minutes, add soy creamer and simmer for another 6 minutes.
8. Let it cool for 5 minutes, serve and enjoy!

Number of servings: 4

Macros (per serving):

Calories: 219.2
Protein: 7.8 g
Carbs: 18.4 g
Fat: 7.9 g

French Onion Soup

Ingredients:

- 1/2 oz. grams of Earth Balance soy free
- 8 oz. white onions, sliced into thin strips
- 13 oz. of Pacific Organic Vegetable Broth low sodium
- 6 1/2 oz. water
- 1/2 tsp. thyme
- Salt and pepper to taste

Directions:

1. Add Earth Balance to stovetop pot and melt on medium heat.
2. Once the pot starts to sizzle, add in the thinly sliced onions.
3. Cook under caramelized or about 15 minutes.
4. Stir constantly under golden brown.
5. Add pepper and thyme and stir and then add in the broth and water.
6. Bring to a boil, reduce heat to a simmer and cook covered for 5 minutes.
7. Take off heat and rest for another 5 minutes, serve and enjoy!

Number of servings: 4

Macros (per serving):

Calories: 52.1
Protein: 0.6 g
Carbs: 6.0 g
Fat: 2.8 g

Lentil Soup

Ingredients:

- 2 cups rinsed lentils
- 1 cup grated carrots
- 1 cup chopped celery
- 1 cup chopped onions
- 3 cloves garlic, minced or crushed
- 1 tbs. paprika
- 1 tsp. chili powder
- 2 tsp. salt
- 1 tsp. black pepper
- 6 cups water

Directions:

1. Rinse lentils and cover with 6 cups water in a large pot, or enough to nearly fill the pot.
2. Cook for about half an hour on medium heat.
3. Next, add all the veggies and seasonings.
4. Cook another half hour to hour, or until all veggies and lentils are soft, on medium heat.
5. Serve and enjoy!

Number of servings: 10

Macros (per serving):

Calories: 63.1
Protein: 4.2 g
Carbs: 11.8 g
Fat: 0.4 g

Stuffed Shells

Ingredients:

Ingredients for the Ricotta

- Tofu, extra firm, 1 block
- Lemon juice from 1/2 lemon
- 1 clove of minced garlic
- 1/4 tsp. salt
- 10 basil leaves
- 2 tsp. olive oil
- 4 tbsp. nutritional yeast

Ingredients for Shells:

- 3 oz. jumbo shells
- 1 1/4 Francesco Rinaldi Tomato & Basil pasta sauce

Directions:

- Preheat oven to 350 degrees F.
- Drain and press the tofu and mush it in a large bowl.
- Add lemon juice, garlic, salt and pepper and chopped basil to the tofu and mush again.
- Add olive oil, stir with a fork and add nutritional yeast. Continue mixing all of the ingredients and then cover the bowl and place in the fridge.
- Boil the pasta shells according to box directions and drain the pasta.
- Pour the majority of the spaghetti sauce into a glass 9"x13" baking pan. Take each of the shells and put a spoonful of ricotta in each.
- Sauce the top of the shells and cover the pan with foil.
- Bake for 25 minutes, take the foil off and bake for another 10 minutes.
- Let cool for ten minutes, serve and enjoy!

Number of servings: 10

Macros (per serving):

Calories: 111.1
Protein: 6.2 g
Carbs: 8.1 g
Fat: 5.8 g

Pumpkin Pancakes (Plant-Based)

Ingredients:

- 2 1/2 cups whole-wheat flour
- 2 1/2 cups water
- 1/2 cup soymilk
- 2 tbsp. baking powder
- 1 tsp. salt
- 1/2 cup mashed, cooked pumpkin
- 1/2 tsp. cinnamon
- 1/4 tsp. nutmeg
- 1/4 tsp. allspice
- 1 tsp. vanilla extract
- 1/2 tsp. baking soda
- 1 tsp. apple cider vinegar

Directions:

1. Put the soymilk and the tsp. vinegar in a bowl, and give it 5 minutes to curdle.
2. After the 5 minutes, add in and stir together the pumpkin, spices, water and soymilk.
3. Add in remaining ingredients and stir until moist.
4. Let the mixture sit for 5 minutes to rise and then lightly stir again.
5. Let rest 5 more minutes and cook them up into 4" pancakes.

Number of servings: 20

Macros (per serving):

Calories: 59.5
Protein: 2.2 g
Carbs: 13.0 g
Fat: 0.4 g

Chickpea Casserole

Ingredients:

- 14 oz. can chickpeas
- 1 tbsp. olive oil
- 14 oz. can tomatoes
- 1 large sliced onion
- 1 tbsp. curry powder
- 2 tbsp. smooth peanut butter
- 1 1/2 oz. of raisins
- 1/2 cup unsweetened apple juice

Directions:

1. Sauté onion in olive oil.
2. Add in chickpeas, curry, canned tomatoes, peanut butter, raisins and apple juice.
3. Cook for 15 minutes.
4. Serve and enjoy!

Number of servings: 4

Macros (per serving):

Calories: 280.5
Protein: 8.8 g
Carbs: 44.6 g
Fat: 9.1 g

Black-Eyed Peas and Tomatoes

Ingredients:

- 3 tbsp. olive oil
- 1 cup of diced onions
- 3-4 cloves of minced garlic
- 2 (10 oz.) pkg. frozen black eyed-peas
- 1 (16 oz.) can of stewed drained tomatoes
- Salt and pepper to taste

Directions:

1. Combine the onions and oil in a small sauté pan with a lid.
2. Cover and cook the onions over low to low-medium heat for 20-30 minutes, stirring occasionally.
3. Add in the peas and the canned tomatoes, including the tomato liquid.
4. Bring to a boil, cover the pan and simmer on low heat for 20 minutes.
5. The peas should be tender and the sauce should have thickened.
6. Season with salt and pepper, serve and enjoy!

Number of servings: 4

Macros (per serving):

Calories: 270.6
Protein: 6.0 g
Carbs: 39.3 g
Fat: 10.9 g

Seitan Fajitas

Ingredients:

- 1 pkg. seitan
- 1 medium chopped onion
- 1 green chopped pepper
- 1/2 cup frozen corn
- 1 tbsp. chili powder
- 1/4 cup water
- 8 corn tortillas
- Salsa to taste

Directions:

1. Cut the seitan into small bite-size pieces and set to the side.
2. Spray a large non-stick skillet with cooking spray.
3. Cook the onion over medium-high heat until soft, and stir occasionally for 5 minutes.
4. Add the corn, green pepper, seitan, chili powder and water to the pan and continue cooking until the peppers are soft.
5. Warm the tortillas and place fajita mixture along with 1 tbsp. of salsa in each tortilla.
6. Serve and enjoy!

Number of servings: 4

Macros (per serving):

Calories: 225.7
Protein: 16.3 g
Carbs: 37.8 g
Fat: 2.8 g

Carrot and Ginger Soup

Ingredients:

- 1 tbsp. olive oil
- 1-1/2 cups diced onions
- 2-3 cloves of minced garlic
- 4 cups fresh chopped carrots
- 1 to 1-1/2 tsp. of grated ginger
- 4 cups vegetable broth
- 1/4 cup orange juice
- 3 cups rice milk
- Salt and pepper to taste

Directions:

1. Sauté the olive oil, onions and garlic in a large pot for 4 minutes.
2. Add in the carrots, ginger and broth and boil for 30 minutes or until the carrots are tender.
3. Puree the mixture in a food processor.
4. Move the mixture to the stove and heat until warm.
5. Add in the orange juice and rice milk, but don't boil it.
6. Add salt and pepper to taste, serve, and enjoy!

Number of servings: 6

Macros (per serving):

Calories: 147.3
Protein: 1.9 g
Carbs: 27.7 g
Fat: 3.6 g

Salad Pasta

Ingredients:

- 4 cups whole-wheat pasta
- 1/4 cup red wine vinegar
- 1/4 cup balsamic vinegar
- 1 tbsp. Dijon mustard
- 1/4 cup extra virgin olive oil
- 2 cloves of minced garlic
- Salt and pepper to taste
- 1/4 cup olives
- 1 small zucchini

Directions:

1. Cook all of the pasta according to package directions and drain it.
2. Drizzle the pasta with half the olive oil to prevent sticking and set aside.
3. Chop olives and zucchini and set them aside.
4. Combine both vinegars, Dijon mustard, remaining olive oil and garlic and whisk them together.
5. Coat pasta with the mixture and add in zucchini and olives. After that, add salt and pepper to taste.
6. Serve and enjoy!

Number of servings: 4

Macros (per serving):

Calories: 368.8
Protein: 7.9 g
Carbs: 45.5 g
Fat: 18.1 g

Banana Peanut Butter Smoothie

Ingredients:

1 large frozen banana
4 tbsp. peanut butter
1 cup rice milk
2 tbsp. ground flax seeds

Directions:

1. Put banana, peanut butter, rice milk and flax seeds in a blender and blend until smooth.
2. Serve and enjoy!

Number of servings: 1

Macros (per serving):

Calories: 684.6
Protein: 21.5 g
Carbs: 73.2 g
Fat: 39.8 g

Pinto Bean Burger

Ingredients:

- 2 cups canned pinto beans
- 1/2 cup Salsa
- 2 tbsp. flax seed meal
- 1 tsp. chili powder
- 1/2 tsp. cumin seed
- 4 oz. crushed tortilla chips

Directions:

1. Preheat oven to 350 degrees F.
2. Combine flax seed meal with 3 tbsp. water. Let it sit for one minute until it forms a paste.
3. In a small mixing bowl, combine all ingredients and mix together until smooth.
4. Form mixture into six patties, and coat both sides with cooking spray.
5. Place patties on a baking sheet, and bake for 20 minutes.
6. Serve and enjoy!

Number of servings: 6

Macros (per serving):

Calories: 166.1
Protein: 6.2 g
Carbs: 26.2 g
Fat: 6.5 g

Spinach Casserole

Ingredients:

- Olive oil for frying
- 1 cup each of chickpeas, pinto and kidney beans
- 1/2 large onion
- 3 cloves of chopped garlic
- 1 cup of thinly sliced red bell peppers
- 10 pitted and chopped black olives
- 2 tins of tomatoes
- 2 tbsp. tomato puree
- 1/2 tsp. salt
- Dash of soy sauce
- Black pepper to taste
- Fresh basil to taste
- 1 bay leaf

Directions:

1. In a large saucepan, add the olive oil and fry the onion then add in the garlic.
2. Toss in the peppers and olives, frying for 5 minutes continuously stirring.
3. Then add in all 3 different kinds of beans.
4. Cook for another 10 minutes, stirring every now and then to make sure the beans don't stick to the bottom of the pan.
5. Add both tins of tomatoes, the tomato paste, salt, soy sauce and bay leaf and place a lid over the saucepan.
6. Simmer on a low heat for an hour to an hour and a half, stirring roughly every 10 minutes.
7. 10 minutes before cooking time is finished, add some chopped basil to taste.
8. Serve and enjoy!

Number of servings: 6

Macros (per serving):

Calories: 205.1
Protein: 8.2 g
Carbs: 31.6 g
Fat: 6.1 g

Stuffed Bell Peppers

Ingredients:

- 6 bell peppers
- 1 can (2 cups) of tomato sauce
- 1 large chopped onion
- 2 cups of sliced mushrooms
- 1 bunch of fresh spinach
- 2 cloves of crushed garlic
- 2 tbsp. of fresh basil
- 1 jalapeño pepper
- 1 cup cooked brown rice
- 1/2 cup of shredded tempeh
- Soy sauce to taste

Directions:

1. Preheat oven to 350 degrees F.
2. Chop all the ingredients minus the bell peppers.
3. Place all the ingredients in a large pot and add olive oil, garlic cloves, fresh basil, jalapeño and onions and cook on high heat for 3 minutes.
4. Add the mushrooms and tempeh and simmer on medium heat for 5 minutes.
5. Toss in the spinach and the rice and cover the pan and turn off the heat to help blend the flavors together.
6. Cut the tops off of the peppers and place the tops to the side.
7. With a spoon, scoop out the seeds from the inside of the bell peppers.
8. Fill the peppers with the mixture and place the tops back on them.
9. Put peppers in a lightly oiled casserole dish and place in oven.
10. Bake the peppers for about 15 minutes.
11. Let cool for 5 minutes, serve, and enjoy!

Number of servings: 6

Macros (per serving):

Calories: 160.6
Protein: 8.8 g
Carbs: 29.9 g
Fat: 2.7 g

Lettuce Wraps

Ingredients:

- 1 large carrot
- 1 spear (5" long) of broccoli
- 1/2 cup of sliced mushrooms
- 1/2 cup of raw chopped onions
- 1/4 head of a small (4" diameter) red cabbage
- 1/2 cup green beans
- 2 tbsp. olive oil
- 2 tbsp. soy sauce
- 4 large leaves of iceberg lettuce

Directions:

1. Chop all of the vegetables.
2. Add 2 tbsp. olive oil to a wok, and turn stove heat on high.
3. Add onions to hot oil and cook for 1 minute.
4. Add remaining vegetables, stir and cover for 1 minute.
5. Repeat until vegetables have reached desired texture.
6. Add soy sauce, cook 30 seconds longer, while stirring to coat the vegetables with the sauce.
7. Pour into bowl and serve with lettuce leaves.

Number of servings: 2

Macros (per serving):

Calories: 212.2
Protein: 3.6 g
Carbs: 20.4 g
Fat: 14.0 g

Potato Leek Soup

Ingredients:

- 6 cups vegetable broth
- 7 small, chopped potatoes
- 3 thinly sliced leeks
- 3-4 cloves of garlic
- A splash of almond milk
- Slat and pepper to taste

Directions:

1. Chop up the potatoes and boil them in a large soup pan with the vegetable broth.
2. Continue to cook potatoes until soft then use a potato masher to mash them up.
3. In a frying pan, sauté the garlic and leeks with a couple tbsp. of water.
4. Once they are soft, add them to the soup pan with the broth and potatoes.
5. Add a splash of almond milk, salt and pepper, and let it all simmer for 10 minutes.

Number of servings: 10

Macros (per serving):

Calories: 120.5
Protein: 3.0 g
Carbs: 27.0 g
Fat: 0.3 g

Bean and Garden Vegetable Soup

Ingredients:

- 6 cups of vegetable broth
- 2 large peeled and diced carrots
- 1 large diced onion
- 4 cloves of minced garlic
- 1/2 head of chopped cabbage
- 1/2 lb. frozen green beans
- 2 tbsp. tomato paste
- 1 1/2 tsp. dried basil and oregano
- 1 tsp. of salt and pepper
- 1 large diced zucchini
- 1, 19 oz. can of dried and rinsed cannellini beans

Directions:

1. Sauté carrots, onion and garlic in a large non-stick pot for 5 minutes.
2. Add all of the remaining ingredients minus the zucchini and cannellini beans and bring to a boil.
3. Cover, reduce heat to medium and simmer for 15 minutes or until the beans are tender.
4. Add the zucchini and cannellini and cook until the zucchini is tender, which will be roughly 7 minutes.

Number of servings: 12

Macros (per serving):

Calories: 75.7
Protein: 3.8 g
Carbs: 15.1 g
Fat: 0.3 g

Beetroot Salad

Ingredients:

- 4 cubed beetroots
- 1 grated carrot
- 1 cubed green apple
- 3 tbsp. of sunflower seeds
- Squeeze of fresh lemon juice
- 2 tsp. olive oil
- Salt and pepper to taste

Directions:

1. Put all of the ingredients in a large bowl and mix well.
2. Serve and enjoy!

Number of servings: 8

Macros (per serving):

Calories: 44.6
Protein: 0.9 g
Carbs: 6.5 g
Fat: 2.1 g

Eggplant Lasagna

Ingredients:

- 1 medium eggplant
- Non-stick Olive Oil Spray
- 2 lasagna noodles
- 1 (14 oz.) block of tofu
- 1/4 cup minced garlic
- 3 cups of traditional spaghetti sauce
- 8 oz. soy cheese

Directions:

1. Boil the lasagna noodles until tender.
2. While the noodles are cooking, cut the eggplant into thin slices.
3. Spray each slice of eggplant with non-stick olive oil spray.
4. Place the eggplant slices on pan and broil them until the pieces are tender.
5. While the eggplant is cooking, put the tofu and garlic in a food processor.
6. Put a few tablespoons of spaghetti sauce in a 9" x 13" baking dish.
7. Place the two lasagna noodles in the bottom of the pan.
8. Spread a few more tablespoons of sauce on top of the noodles.
9. Spread some of the tofu mixture on top of the sauce.
10. Sprinkle some soy cheese on the top of the tofu mixture.
11. Layer some of the eggplant on top of the cheese.
12. Repeat the previous 3 steps (8-11) until all of the eggplant has been used.
13. Place the remaining sauce, tofu and cheese on top of the last layer of eggplant.

14. Bake at 350 degrees F until the soy cheese is melted.
15. Cut the lasagna into 12 equal slices.
16. Let cool for 10 minutes, serve and enjoy!

Number of servings: 12

Macros (per serving):

Calories: 130.5
Protein: 9.8 g
Carbs: 16.3 g
Fat: 4.7 g

Gumbo with Collard Greens

Ingredients:

- 1 bunch of chopped collard greens
- 1/2 tbsp. of olive oil
- 1 cup of chopped onions
- 1 chopped green bell pepper
- 3/4 cup of sliced celery
- 2 tsp. of minced garlic
- 1 cup of chopped tomatoes
- 1/2 tbsp. of ground thyme
- 3 cubes (makes 6 cups) of low sodium vegetable bouillon
- 6 cups of water
- 1 can (15 oz.) of drained red kidney beans
- 1 tsp. of Tabasco sauce
- Salt and pepper to taste

Directions:

1. Prepare the bouillon by dissolving in boiling water and set it aside.
2. Cook the collard greens in a pot of boiling water for 7 minutes, and drain the pot and set it aside.
3. Spray large pot with non-stick cooking spray. Heat the oil in same pot over medium heat.
4. Add the onion, bell pepper, celery and garlic to the pot, and cook it covered for 5 minutes, occasionally stirring.
5. Toss in the tomatoes and thyme.
6. Add the bouillon broth and salt and pepper to taste.
7. Simmer on low heat for 30 minutes, and stir occasionally.
8. Add in the collards, beans and Tabasco sauce.
9. Taste to adjust the seasoning and cook 10 to 15 minutes longer.

10. Serve and enjoy!

Number of servings: 6

Macros (per serving):

Calories: 147.9
Protein: 8.2 g
Carbs: 23.6 g
Fat: 3.6 g

Italian Skillet (Plant-Based)

Ingredients:

- 1/2 tbsp. extra virgin olive oil
- 3 links of sliced Tofurky Italian Sausage
- 1/2 cup of diced onion
- 2 large sliced zucchini squash
- 1 (14.5 oz.) can of diced tomatoes w/ basil, garlic, and oregano

Directions:

1. Brown the sausage slices in the olive oil with the onions over medium high heat. Next, add the zucchini, and sweat it for 2 minutes.
2. Throw in the tomatoes and cover.
3. Simmer for 15 minutes.
4. Serve and enjoy!

Number of servings: 4

Macros (per serving):

Calories: 276.7
Protein: 23.4 g
Carbs: 20.2 g
Fat: 11.6 g

Tofu Cubes with BBQ

Ingredients:

- 1 block of tofu
- 1 cup of vegan barbecue sauce
- 1 cup of water
- 2 tbsp. of soy sauce
- 1 tbsp. of hot sauce
- 2 tbsp. of granulated sugar
- 2 tbsp. of olive oil

Directions:

1. Dice tofu into cubes about the size of small cubes.
2. Heat oil in frying pan and add tofu.
3. Sauté the tofu on medium until it turn golden.
4. Toss in the ingredients.
5. Stir in the sauces to the mixture.
6. Keep cooking on medium until the sauce has thickened.

Number of servings: 4

Macros (per serving):

Calories: 207.7
Protein: 14.4 g
Carbs: 14.1 g
Fat: 11.6 g

Breakfast Scramble

Ingredients:

- 1/4 cup of raw red onion
- 1 1/2 cup of green bell peppers
- 2 cups of fresh mushrooms
- 1 med. head of raw cauliflower (5-6" dia.)
- 1 tsp. ground turmeric
- 1/4 tsp. of red pepper flakes
- 3 cloves of garlic
- 2 tbsp. low sodium soy sauce
- 2 tbsp. of yeast flakes
- Salt and pepper to taste

Directions:

1. Put the onions, peppers and mushrooms in a skillet over medium heat, and cook for 7-8 minutes.
2. Add 1 to 2 tbsp. of water to keep from sticking.
3. Add in the cauliflower, and cook for another 5 minutes.
4. Add seasonings, soy sauce and yeast.
5. Cook for 5 more minutes, serve and enjoy!

Number of servings: 6

Macros (per serving):

Calories: 64.6
Protein: 5.1 g
Carbs: 12.7 g
Fat: 0.9 g

Plant-Based Breakfast

Ingredients:

- 1 cup of warm water
- 2 cups of coffee
- 1 tbsp. coconut oil
- 2 tbsp. (15 grams) NutriBiotic brown rice vanilla protein powder
- 12 raw almonds

Directions:

1. Using a blender and a deep container that holds at least 2 cups, blend the hot coffee, coconut oil and brown rice protein powder.
2. Pour this mixture into your coffee cup, and drink this while you eat the 12 almonds.
3. Pour another cup of coffee into the same cup to get the rest of the protein powder that may have stuck to the bottom.

Number of servings: 1

Macros (per serving):

Calories: 282.8
Protein: 15.8 g
Carbs: 7.1 g
Fat: 21.1 g

Plant-Based Chocolate Ice Cream

Ingredients:

- 1, 15oz can of coconut milk
- 2 tbsp. xylitol
- 2 tbsp. unsweetened cocoa powder
- 1/2 cup unsweetened plain almond milk

Directions:

1. Mix together all ingredients until thoroughly combined.
2. Move the mixture to a container and seal with a lid.
3. Put mixture in freezer for about 2-3 hours, and stir the mixture every half-hour.
4. Serve and enjoy!

Number of servings: 6

Macros (per serving):

Calories: 159.5
Protein: 2.0 g
Carbs: 3.4 g
Fat: 15.8 g

Vegan Coconut Truffles

Ingredients:

- 1 tbsp. raw organic coconut oil
- 1 tbsp. unsweetened shredded coconut
- 1/2 tsp. xylitol
- 1 tbsp. cocoa powder

Directions:

1. Blend together the coconut oil, shredded coconut and xylitol.
2. Refrigerate until set, which should be roughly 10 minutes.
3. Cut into 2 cubes or roll into 2 balls.
4. Next roll the cubes/balls in the cocoa powder.
5. Serve and enjoy!

Number of servings: 2

Macros (per serving):

Calories: 113.8
Protein: 1.0 g
Carbs: 3.2 g
Fat: 11.7 g

Guacamole

Ingredients:

- 4 avocadoes
- 1 tub fresh salsa, pico de gallo style, including vinegar brine
- 3/4 cup chopped fresh cilantro
- 1/4 - 1/2 tbsp. salt
- 1/4 tbsp. chopped garlic

Directions:

1. Put all of the ingredients in a blender and mix together.
2. Place guacamole in a bowl and cover with wax paper to prevent browning and then seal the bowl.
3. Allow guacamole to sit at least 1 hour before serving.

Number of servings: 16

Macros (per serving):

Calories: 79.1
Protein: 0.8 g
Carbs: 4.7 g
Fat: 6.8 g

Mushroom Stroganoff

Ingredients:

- 2 tsp. fresh thyme
- 1 tsp. of rosemary
- 50 Portobello mushrooms
- 4 fluid oz. white wine
- 2 servings (1 stalk) of green onion
- 4 cloves of garlic
- 16 oz. of whole-wheat linguine
- 16 tbsp. tofu sour cream
- 1 tbsp. parsley

Directions:

1. Cook the green onion over medium heat for 8 minutes.
2. In a separate pot, cook the noodles over medium heat.
3. Add 2 tbsp. of water to prevent the onion from sticking to the pan.
4. Add in the garlic and thyme, and cook for 1 minute.
5. Add in and stir the rosemary and Portobello mushrooms, cooking for 10 minutes and stirring occasionally.
6. Add in the wine, stirring and cooking over low-medium heat for 20 minutes.
7. When the stroganoff is finished cooking, add and stir in the sour cream.
8. Add in the cooked noodles (garnished with parsley) and toss well.
9. Combine all ingredients in a blender and puree until smooth and creamy.
10. Serve and enjoy!

Number of servings: 4

Macros (per serving):

Calories: 646.5
Protein: 19.1 g
Carbs: 107.7 g
Fat: 13.3 g

Avocado Sandwich

Ingredients:

- 1/2 of an avocado, skin and seeds removed
- 2 slices of vegan bread
- 1 leaf of romaine lettuce
- 2 tbsp. of Cilantro salad dressing

Directions:

1. Place all of the ingredients in between the 2 slices of bread.
2. Serve and enjoy!

Number of servings: 1

Macros (per serving):

Calories: 355.9
Protein: 10.9 g
Carbs: 40.7 g
Fat: 17.9 g

"Egg" Sandwich

Ingredients:

- 1/5 block of extra firm tofu
- 2 oz. of Light Life Gimme Lean Sausage
- 1/4 inch thick slice of an anise bulb
- 2 slices of complete protein style bread
- 1 tbsp. of ketchup
- 1/2 tsp. of tumeric
- 1/2 tsp. of cumin
- 1/2 tsp. of cayenne pepper

Directions:

1. Coat a frying pan with Canola oil spray.
2. Cut the tofu into two slices.
3. Form sausage into a thin patty roughly the size of the bread slices.
4. Place the patty, tofu slices and anise slice into the pan.
5. Sprinkle the spices onto the tofu.
6. Grill for 4 minutes and then turn over and repeat.
7. Place between lightly toasted bread and add ketchup.
8. Serve and enjoy!

Number of servings: 1

Macros (per serving):

Calories: 264.3
Protein: 21.9 g
Carbs: 29.4 g
Fat: 6.4 g

Corn Chowder

Ingredients:

- 1 1/2 tbsp. of butter substitute
- 1 tbsp. of soy based bacon bits
- 1/2 cup of chopped yellow onion
- 1/2 cup of chopped carrots
- 1/2 cup of chopped celery
- 3 ears (app. 2 cups) of sweet corn with the kernels removed
- 1 bay leaf
- 4 cups of light soymilk
- 2 medium diced and peeled turnips
- 1/2 cup of chopped red bell pepper
- Salt and pepper to taste
- 1/2 tsp. of fresh thyme leaves
- 1/2 cup TVP
- 8 tbsp. of nutritional yeast

Directions:

1. In a large saucepan, melt the butter substitute over medium heat.
2. Next, add in the soy based bacon bits and sauté until flavor released (roughly 1-2 minutes).
3. Add in the onion and sauté for 4-5 minutes until soft.
4. Throw in the carrots and celery and cook for an additional 5 minutes.
5. Add in the corn to the saucepan.
6. After that, add in the soymilk and the bay leaf.
7. Bring to a boil and reduce heat to a bare simmer.
8. Cover the pot and cook on low heat for 30 minutes.
9. Raise the heat; add in the turnips, red pepper and salt and pepper to taste.
10. Bring to a simmer and reduce the heat again to maintain a simmer for 12 minutes.

11. Raise the heat. Add in the removed corn kernels, thyme, TVP and yeast.
12. Bring to a boil and make sure the yeast is mixed in well.
13. Reduce the heat and simmer for 5 minutes, serve and enjoy!

Number of servings: 4

Macros (per serving):

Calories: 277.2
Protein: 22.9 g
Carbs: 37.3 g
Fat: 6.3 g

Tomato and Tofu Soup

Ingredients:

- 5 large peeled and cored ripe tomatoes
- 1/2 pkg. (16 oz.) medium tofu
- 2 tsp. of vegetable stock
- 1 finely chopped celery stalk
- 1 medium finely chopped onion
- 1 tsp. of lemon juice
- 1 tbsp. of parsley
- 1 tsp. of salt
- 1 tsp. of pepper

Directions:

1. Puree the tomatoes with the tofu.
2. Put the tomatoes and tofu in a pot with the rest of the ingredients.
3. Cook for 20 minutes or until tender, serve and enjoy.

Number of servings: 4

Macros (per serving):

Calories: 248.2
Protein: 21.1 g
Carbs: 23.7 g
Fat: 10.9 g

Raisin Pumpkin Muffins

Ingredients:

- 1 cup rice flour
- 3/4 all-purpose GF flour
- 1 1/4 cup sugar
- 1 1/4 tbsp. baking powder
- 1 tsp. ground cinnamon
- 1/2 tsp. nutmeg
- 1/2 tsp. ground ginger
- 1/4 tsp. allspice
- 1/8 tsp. ground cloves
- 1 cup cooked mashed pumpkin
- 1/2 cup soymilk
- 1/2 cup vegetable oil
- 2 tbsp. molasses
- 1/2 cup raisins
- Salt to taste

Directions:

1. Preheat oven to 400 degrees F and grease the muffin tin.
2. Cover raisins in hot water and set to the side.
3. Sift together all of the dry ingredients.
4. In a separate bowl, whisk together all of the wet ingredients.
5. Pour the wet ingredient mixture into the dry and mix together.
6. Drain the raisins and gently fold them in.
7. Fill muffin tins 2/3 full.
8. Bake for 25 minutes or until toothpick comes out clean.
9. Let cool for 5 minutes, serve and enjoy!

Number of servings: 13

Macros (per serving):

Calories: 255.5
Protein: 2.2 g
Carbs: 43.3 g
Fat: 8.9 g

Broccoli Salad

Ingredients:

- 4 cups of freshly chopped broccoli
- 1/4 cup of fresh finely chopped onion
- 1/4 cup of packed raisins
- 1/4 cup fat free mayonnaise substitute
- 1 tsp. of vinegar
- 2 packets of Stevia

Directions:

1. Mix the mayonnaise, vinegar and sweetener together in a bowl.
2. Mix broccoli, onions and raisins together in a bowl.
3. Toss the salad with dressing, serve and enjoy!

Number of servings: 4

Macros (per serving):

Calories: 69.6
Protein: 3.1 g
Carbs: 13.7 g
Fat: 0.4 g

Chapter 10: Frequently Asked Questions

I'm worried that I won't be able to get enough protein to meet my macro needs. What should I do?

Not being able to get enough protein is certainly one of the most common worries people have about a plant-based diet. The reality is that you can easily get enough protein if you plan ahead wisely and eat the right foods such as the following:

- Hemp
- Quinoa
- Tofu
- Lentils
- Nuts
- Tempeh
- Beans

Is a Plant-Based Diet the Healthiest Diet There Is?

This is a tricky question to answer. The reality is that there are many diets out there that strive to have you eating more natural, unprocessed foods. This, of course, is the ultimate goal because to get and stay healthy you need to eat clean foods. A plant-based diet does stand out by eliminating all animal based foods, whereas other healthy diets don't cut out all animal foods. However, it's hard to pinpoint a specific diet and say it's inherently the best because of X, Y and Z. Rest assured though, you'll become way healthier by starting a plant-based diet.

How much weight should I lift during the workouts?

Lift as much weight as you possibly can for the given rep range. Initially, you won't know how much weight to use so you'll have to take your best guess. For example, let's say you're doing bench press for 8 reps. You think you can lift around 150 pounds for that many reps, but on your first set you easily complete 10 reps.

This means the weight is too light and you need to increase it for the next set. On the next set you lift 165 pounds and struggle to complete the 8th rep. This is what you want to happen and it means you've found a good weight to use. Once you can complete all 3 sets for 8 reps with 165 pounds, move up to 170 the next time you bench press. If you can't complete 8 reps for all 3 sets, stick with 165 until you can. Here's an example:

Workout 1: Bench Press with 165 pounds
Set 1: 8 reps
Set 2: 8 reps
Set 3: 7 reps

Because you only completed 7 reps on the last set, stick with 165 for the next workout—

Workout 2: Bench Press with 165 pounds
Set 1: 8 reps
Set 2: 8 reps
Set 3: 8 reps

Because you completed all 3 sets for 8 reps, move up to 170 on your next workout with bench press.

Note: It's better to use a weight that's too heavy and miss a rep or two than it is to use a weight that's too light and leave some reps in the tank. For example, it's better to do 170 pounds and only complete 6 reps instead of 8 opposed to using 155 pounds and stopping at 8 reps even though you could've easily done more reps.

How Fast Should I Lose Weight?

The more weight you have to lose, the faster the rate at which you can lose the weight. For example, if you have 50+ pounds to lose, you can lose weight at a rate of 2 pounds or more per week. If you only have 5 pounds to lose, then you'll lose weight at a rate of .5 pound per week.

For most people, losing 1 pound per week is the sweet spot. You'll be creating an average caloric deficit of 500 calories daily. At this pace, you'll be losing weight fairly quickly and you won't be miserable all of the time from a complete lack of calories.

How much water should I drink on a daily basis?

Your body is made up of about 60% water, so it's important to consume water for several reasons:

- Helps keep your joints and ligaments fluid, which can help prevent injury
- Helps control your caloric intake
- Flushes out toxins
- Improves skin quality
- Improves kidney function
- Improves your focus

Many people recommend that you should drink 1 gallon of water per day. This is a blanket answer that doesn't meet individual needs. This recommendation would have a 100-

pound woman drinking the same amount of water as a 200-pound man. Absurd!

Other health experts advise drinking eight 8-ounce glasses (64 ounces total) of water a day. But again 64 ounces isn't going to be enough for most people. What should you do then? I don't keep track of my water intake—I go by how I feel and the color of my urine.

Your body's own thirst mechanism will be accurate in telling you if you need more water. If you feel thirsty, go drink some water. If not, you're probably ok. You can also use the color of your urine to judge how hydrated you are. If your urine is yellow, then you should drink more water. If it's clear, then you should be good to go. This keeps things simple and it's one less thing you have to keep track of.

How Do I Motivate Myself to Go to the Gym?

Finding the motivation to go to the gym or eat right can be hard. No matter who you are, there will be times when you don't feel like working out. Having that feeling is ok, but you can't let it control you. There will be times when you'll have to do it anyway, even when you don't feel like it.

That's what will ultimately separate a long-term successful fitness journey from failing at it. I do have some tips to help you out along the way, however:

Tip #1: Focus on Gradual Improvements

Many people make fitness an all-or-nothing game. They tell themselves that they'll workout 5 days a week and eat clean 100% of the time for the rest of their lives. Let's say you workout only 4 days one week. Are you a failure?

Of course not. You still worked out 4 days, but in your mind you are because you failed to reach 5 workouts. You make it

111

hard to celebrate any small successes that you do have because the standards are too high.

Instead, focus on making smaller, more gradual improvements, and celebrate any successes you have along the way. For example, start off with a goal to only workout 2 days per week if it's been years since you've last worked out. Once you achieve that goal, you'll feel good about yourself, and you can move up to working out 3 days per week and so on.

Tip #2: Action Leads Motivation

People think they have to get the inspiration or motivation from somewhere in order to take the action necessary to workout. The reverse of that is actually true. You need to start by taking an action no matter how small. And once you get started, you'll likely want to continue on with what you're doing.

When I think about everything I have to do to workout: put my gym clothes on, drive to the gym, workout with a bunch of grueling exercises, drive back and shower—I start to make up silly excuses as to why I should skip this time. Instead, I'll tell myself to do just one exercise when I get to the gym and not pressure myself to do anything more. After I finish that first exercise, it's always easier for me to finish the rest of the workout.

You just have to get started. Try this out for any healthy habit you want to start. For example, if you want to start flossing your teeth, tell yourself you'll only floss one tooth and don't pressure yourself to do anything more than that! This trick might sound silly, but it works because it's all about getting started. Try it out; see if you can floss just one tooth.

Tip #3: Put Your Own Money on the Line

Money is a very powerful motivator. And you can use your own money to motivate yourself to start working out more. Here's what you're going to do—give someone a good amount of money. Not $20, but something that would actually hurt you—$100, $200, $500 or whatever you can't afford to lose.

Then tell your friend that if you don't go to the gym 3 days this week, they get to keep the money. When you give up the money in the first place, you'll fight to get it back. This is much different than telling yourself you'll give the money to someone after you miss your workouts.

It's too easy to make an excuse and not give away the money. Give the money up in the first place, and make sure your friend actually holds you accountable to it. This is by far the best way to get motivation to workout. There's a real cost involved if you don't comply. You'll either get ripped or go broke trying.

Conclusion

Thanks for reading this book all the way to the end! I firmly believe that it's truly possible for you to achieve a healthy and good-looking body that you're proud of by following the nutritional and training advice outlined in this book. Getting fit isn't easy, but it's worth it. Stay strong and persist even when you mess up, and you'll succeed in the long run.

Finally, if you have any questions, please be sure to email me at thomas@rohmerfitness.com. I'd be more than happy to answer any questions that you have!

Sources

(1) https://www.cdc.gov/nchs/fastats/obesity-overweight.htm

(2) https://www.cdc.gov/heartdisease/facts.htm

(3) https://www.ncbi.nlm.nih.gov/pubmed/24687909

(4) https://www.ncbi.nlm.nih.gov/pubmed/24871675

(5) http://journals.plos.org/plosone/article?id=10.1371/journal.pone.0000698

(6) https://www.epa.gov/ghgemissions/sources-greenhouse-gas-emissions

(7) http://usda.mannlib.cornell.edu/usda/nass/LiveSlau//2010s/2017/LiveSlau-08-24-2017.pdf

(8) https://www.ncbi.nlm.nih.gov/pubmed/25592014

(9) https://www.arthritisresearchuk.org/arthritis-information/conditions/osteoporosis/who-gets-it.aspx

(10) https://www.ncbi.nlm.nih.gov/pubmed/11600749

(11) https://www.webmd.com/heart/metabolic-syndrome/metabolic-syndrome-what-is-it#1

(12) https://www.ncbi.nlm.nih.gov/pubmcd/11518143

(13) http://www.apa.org/research/action/multitask.aspx

(14) https://www.ncbi.nlm.nih.gov/pubmed/22825659

(15) https://www.ncbi.nlm.nih.gov/pubmed/23521346

(16) https://en.wikipedia.org/wiki/Television_consumption

(17) https://www.cbsnews.com/news/cdc-80-percent-of-american-adults-dont-get-recommended-exercise/

(18) http://www.thewalkingsite.com/10000steps.html

(19) http://naturalsociety.com/the-1-best-way-to-cleanse-the-lymphatic-system/

(20) http://fortune.com/2016/01/15/powerball-lottery-winners/

*Recipes courtesy of Sparkrecipes.com

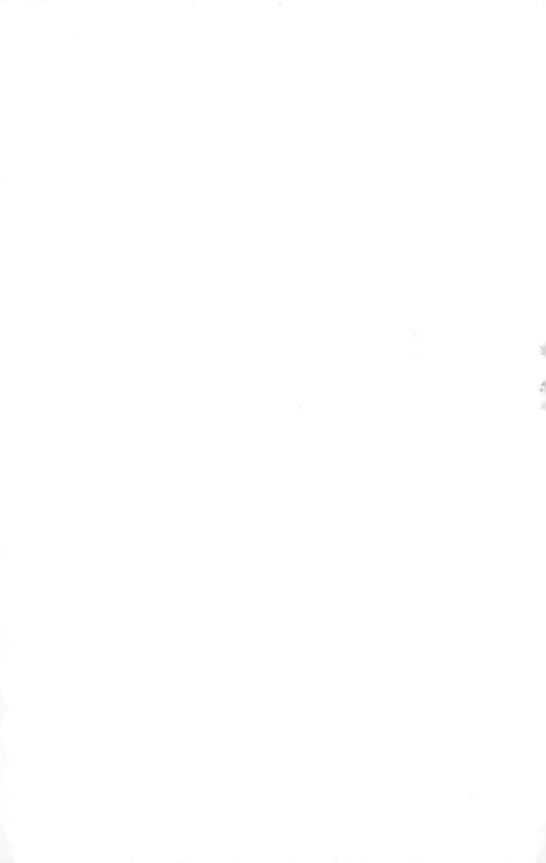

21986862R00067

Printed in Poland
by Amazon Fulfillment
Poland Sp. z o.o., Wrocław